Physiology of the Gastrointestinal Tract

Physiology of the Gastrointestinal Tract

Edited by

GRAEME DUTHIE, MD (Hons), FRCSEd,
Reader in Surgery, Castle Hill Hospital, Cottingham

and

ANGELA GARDINER, BSc (Hons), MPhil,
Clinical Physiologist, Castle Hill Hospital, Cottingham

W

WHURR PUBLISHERS
LONDON AND PHILADELPHIA

© 2004 Whurr Publishers Ltd

First Published 2004
Whurr Publishers Ltd
19b Compton Terrace, London N1 2UN, England and
325 Chestnut Street, Philadelphia PA19106, USA

British Library Cataloguing in Publication Data

A catalogue record for this book is available from the
British Library.

ISBN 1 86156 276 4

Printed and bound in the UK by Athenaeum Press Limited,
Gateshead, Tyne & Wear.

Contents

Contributors

Ged R Avery, Consultant Radiologist, Castle Hill Hospital, Cottingham

Patrick J Byrne, Lecturer in Gastrointestinal Physiology, Department of Surgery, Trinity College Dublin at St James's Hospital, Dublin

Simon Dexter, Consultant Surgeon, Leeds General Infirmary, Leeds

David F Evans, Gastrointestinal Physiology Unit, St Bartholomew's and Royal London Hospital, London

Ridzuan Farouk, Consultant Surgeon, Department of Colorectal Surgery, Royal Berkshire and Battle Hospitals, Reading

Angela Gardiner, Clinical Physiologist, Castle Hill Hospital, Cottingham

Geetinder Kaur, Research Fellow, Castle Hill Hospital, Cottingham

Amanda Roy, Clinical Scientist, Motility Unit, Addenbrooke's Hospital, Cambridge

Spike Smilgin Humphreys, Clinical Nurse Specialist, GI Clinical Physiology, John Radcliffe Hospital, Oxford

Lynne Smith, Chief Clinical Physiologist, GI Investigation, Northern General Hospital, Sheffield

Herr Hsin Tsai, Consultant Gastroenterologist, Castle Hill Hospital, Cottingham

JP Vasani, Specialist Registrar, Castle Hill Hospital, Cottingham

Michael ER Williamson, Consultant Colorectal Surgeon, Royal United Hospital, Bath

Etsuro Yazaki, Manager and Honorary Lecturer GI Science, Gastrointestinal Physiology Unit, St Bartholomew's and Royal London Hospital, London

Preface

Both upper and lower gastrointestinal (GI) physiology have come of age over the last few years, both in the extent of their use in clinical medicine and in the training of technicians and nurse practitioners to undertake physiological assessment. State registration is here now for GI physiologists and, in the past, there have been no good books aimed at GI physiologists themselves or nurse practitioners who have an interest in undertaking the physiology that covers both technical and clinical aspects of the job. This book will, it is hoped, fill this gap and be of interest to those groups; it should also be extremely useful to those doctors in gastroenterology and surgery who need to know about GI physiological assessment.

We hope that this book fills all those needs, but moreover we hope that it is easy to read and will explain why this sub-specialty area is becoming more popular and more important.

Angela Gardiner and Graeme Duthie

Chapter 1

Indications for gastrointestinal physiological assessment

Patrick J Byrne

There are many indications for physiological assessment of the upper and lower gastrointestinal (GI) tract. Many of these are well developed in clinical practice. In addition to these indications, those for less common types of GI investigations such as oesophageal manometry, anorectal manometry and biliary manometry are discussed, to give an overview of the range of facilities available for GI physiological assessment.

Oesophageal manometry

Oesophageal manometry can be useful in the diagnosis and/or management of gastro-oesophageal reflux, dysphagia and chest pain of oesophageal origin. It is also useful in defining pathology extrinsic from the oesophagus, in which abnormal manometry may be just one component.

Manometry should be carried out by an experienced operator. Stationary manometry is the most widely used technique while ambulatory manometry, although more physiological, is not used routinely. The availability of computerized systems, with automatic analysis, has largely replaced pen recorder systems. However, reliance on automatic analysis alone can result in misinterpretation of data. Operator intervention is often required to classify events manually. The best manometry software should allow for both manual and automatic analysis. Ambulatory differs from stationary manometry in that it is usually carried out over 24 hours and together with pH monitoring. A typical ambulatory system will include four channels of pressure and one or two pH channels. There are no accepted normal values for ambulatory data, although this technique is potentially useful in documenting motility changes during symptoms that are less likely to be reproduced during a short study in an unphysiological setting such as the manometry laboratory.

Parameters are posture dependent[1]. Amplitudes of contraction and sphincter pressure are higher when the patient is supine compared with semi-recumbent or upright positions. Perfusion manometry investigations should always be carried out in the supine position because it is difficult to compensate for hydrostatic errors if used in the upright position. On the other hand, microtransducer systems will give accurate values for all postures. As technique varies between investigators, care should be taken when comparing results from different centres.

Resting lower oesophageal sphincter (LOS) measurement is not difficult, but many different methods of interpretation are used. Different values will be obtained depending on the technique, e.g. continuous pull through or stationary pull through. Resting pressure for stationary pull through is usually taken as the measurement of inherent muscle tone, which is end-expiratory pressure (Figure 1.1), but some users specify that this measurement should be at the point of respiratory reversal. If automatic computer sphincter analysis is used, then the value obtained will be mean sphincter pressure, which will be different again. End-inspiratory pressure, on the other hand, is a measurement of the total oesophageal–gastric junction pressure. The lower oesophageal sphincter shows marked asymmetry. Using a four-channel perfused catheter with 90° orientation, it is obvious that different pressures are measured in different orientations. With this configuration and perfused stationary manometry, resting pressure should be calculated as end-expiratory pressure at the point of respiratory reversal, averaged over four channels.

The point of respiratory reversal for a sphincter in normal position is when the catheter sensor transverses the diaphragm. Under normal conditions, the sphincter is approximately 4 cm long. The crural diaphragm encircles the proximal 2 cm of the sphincter. Therefore, about 50 per cent of the sphincter length lies below the diaphragm and is exposed to intra-abdominal pressure, the proximal part of the sphincter being exposed to intrathoracic pressure. This can be demonstrated on a sphincter trace by examining the respiratory excursions that are in phase with chest wall movement (higher pressure with inspiration) when the pressure sensor is below the diaphragm, and out of phase when

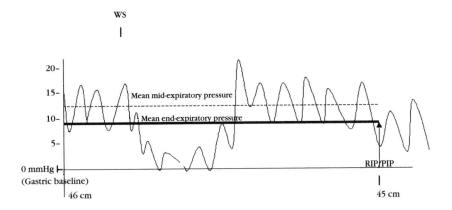

Figure 1.1 Illustration of end-expiratory pressure of lower oesophageal sphincter.

exposed to intrathoracic pressure (lower pressures on inspiration). In patients with a hiatus hernia, respiratory reversal may not correspond with crossing the sphincter if the stomach has moved up into the chest.

Gastro-oesophageal reflux disease

Manometry alone cannot reliably predict clinically significant gastro-oesophageal reflux (GOR). However, the manometric detection of the sphincter is essential for accurate placement of the pH probe for ambulatory pH monitoring. Studies[2] have shown that there is a significant error in placing the pH probe using information from endoscopy or sphincter detection by pH change alone. It is now common practice to include lower sphincter identifiers in commercial pH monitors, which allow the user to locate the LOS by measuring the pressure during a sphincter pull through, thus identifying the position of the proximal border of the sphincter. Sphincter identifiers give limited information about motility because they are single channel only. A full oesophageal manometry investigation requires a minimum of four pressure channels.

Impaired peristalsis or LOS dysfunction is a poor predictor of reflux[3]. Patients with severe reflux disease do have low sphincter pressures and reduced amplitude of contraction, resulting in poor oesophageal clearance. However, it is not known whether or not these changes are secondary to oesophagitis. The anti-reflux mechanism is much more complicated than first thought[4]. The sphincter mechanism not only includes the intrinsic smooth muscle of the distal oesophagus, but also is under the influence of the skeletal muscle of the crural diaphragm. Measurement of oesophagogastric junction pressure is a combination of inherent muscle tone and the pressure exerted by the crural diaphragm during inspiration. Low sphincter pressure alone, as measured by manometry, is not a good predictor of reflux, although an incompetent LOS is widely accepted as intrinsic tone less than 5 mmHg. Reflux occurs most frequently during transient lower oesophageal sphincter relaxations (TLOSRs) and this can occur even when there appears to be adequate muscle tone. For reflux to occur by this mechanism, simultaneous relaxation of the crural diaphragm is necessary. Sphincter manometry using sleeve devices is particularly helpful in documenting TLOSRs. However, a prolonged study is required which should include a 2-hour period after eating.

Laparoscopic surgery is now considered as a reasonable alternative to medical therapy for GOR disease (GORD). It has the advantages of reduced hospital stay compared with open surgery, and patients are back to normal activity more quickly. There is therefore some debate about the most appropriate preoperative and postoperative assessment[5]. Manometry has a role in the preoperative assessment of these patients, particularly if there is some uncertainty about the diagnosis of GORD. Manometry also helps to exclude primary motility disturbances such as achalasia or diffuse oesophageal spasm, which if present would only be compounded by anti-reflux surgery[6]. Impaired peristalsis or ineffective motility has been suggested as a contraindication to anti-reflux surgery. However, the evidence for this is sparse, others suggesting[7] that 'Nissen fundoplication may be safely performed in those patients who are genuinely refractory to vigorous medical treatment regardless of the subtleties of preoperative manometry or pH recording.' The position statement of the American Gastroenterological Association[7] on oesophageal manometry states that 'Manometry is possibly indicated for the pre-operative assessment of peristaltic function in patients being considered for anti-reflux surgery.' Ineffective motility preoperatively may influence the type of anti-reflux surgery carried out[8]. The incomplete wrap or Belsey operation is favoured by some[9]. Routine postoperative assessment should also include manometry; there is evidence that the increase in sphincter pressure after fundoplication persists for more than 7 years in those patients assessed at 3–6 months after surgery. Postoperative transient dysphagia occurs in a significant percentage of patients after fundoplication, frequently disappearing after about 3 months. However, there is no evidence that there is a relationship between the preoperative ineffective motility and the postoperative dysphagia.

Primary motility disorders

Achalasia

Achalasia may present with clinical symptoms such as dysphagia, for both solids and liquids, regurgitation, weight loss and chest pain; the radiological features may also be characteristic, but manometry remains the most reliable method of establishing a diagnosis. Infiltration of the lower oesophageal myenteric plexus by a tumour of the cardia may also resemble achalasia, and is termed 'pseudoachalasia'. Care should be taken to ensure that endoscopy has ruled out the presence of a tumour in order to exclude the possibility of mistaking pseudoachalasia for achalasia. Achalasia is characterized by the absence of peristalsis in the smooth muscle of the oesophageal body, incomplete relaxation of the LOS in response to swallowing, and a normal or high resting LOS pressure. The resting pressure in the oesophageal body is often higher than gastric pressure, possibly as a result of stasis of food, fluid or air[10]. This elevation is accentuated during eating and can reach pressures in excess of 100 mmHg. A small number of patients exhibit vigorous achalasia, a variation in which non-peristaltic contractions of more normal amplitude are seen. It is sometimes difficult to measure relaxation of the sphincter reliably using a side-hole perfusion catheter technique. The longitudinal muscle in the oesophagus shortens during swallowing and the sensor may slip out of the sphincter, although an experienced operator can usually adjust for this movement. A sleeve device is more reliable than a side-hole measurement for sphincter relaxation, but sleeve catheters are frequently expensive and of larger diameter than the routine four-channel perfusion catheter.

Treatment of achalasia can be medical or surgical, the intention with either treatment being to reduce the LOS pressure and restore the sphincter function. Traditional medical treatment consists of balloon dilatation, but other treatments such as botulinum toxin injections are becoming popular. Surgical myotomy for achalasia gives good symptomatic relief. However, post-treatment manometry usually shows that peristalsis remains absent from the smooth muscle of the oesophageal body. The main manometric post-treatment finding in patients who have symptomatic relief is reduced LOS pressure.

Diffuse oesophageal spasm

The diagnosis of diffuse oesophageal spasm is based on manometric findings of simultaneous oesophageal body contractions after pharyngeal contraction, in the presence of normal lower oesophageal function. The simultaneous contractions are not present in all swallows, but should be present in more than 30 per cent of them. The contractions are often multi-peaked and prolonged. The main differentiating feature between diffuse spasm and vigorous achalasia is normal sphincter function. Many names have been given to this disorder – mainly based on radiological appearance – including corkscrew oesophagus, rosary bead oesophagus, functional diverticula, segmental spasm, elevator oesophagus and knuckle buster[11]. Patients may present with central chest pain and/or dysphagia. Referrals are often from the cardiology service because the features of this condition often mimic the type of pain experienced with angina pectoris associated with myocardial ischaemia. Oesophageal spasms are sometimes induced by emotion or food. However, some patients have these attacks only rarely, making the diagnosis difficult[12]. Provocation tests such as balloon inflation or administration of a cholinesterase inhibitor (e.g. edrophonium) may be helpful in provoking the abnormality. Manometry may be used to see if the provoked pain is the result of oesophageal spasm although manometric abnormalities can be present when the patient is asymptomatic, and even when symptoms are reproduced using provocation tests there is poor correlation between symptoms and worsening of the manometric abnormality.

Nutcracker oesophagus

Nutcracker oesophagus is also known as 'symptomatic oesophageal peristalsis'. The proportion of patients with this diagnosis has increased more as patients with angina-like chest pain of non-cardiac origin are investigated for oesophageal disease. Nutcracker oesophagus accounts for 28–43 per cent of motor disorders in patients with non-cardiac, angina-like chest pain. It is therefore the most common disorder encountered in the manometry laboratory.

Symptoms of this condition include non-cardiac chest pain, frequently associated with exertion, and patients sometimes have dysphagia. Manometric diagnosis of nutcracker oesophagus usually shows the sphincter pressure to be normal or hypertensive. The main abnormality is excessively high propagated pressure waves with amplitudes of contraction in excess of 180 mmHg in the distal oesophagus. This amplitude threshold refers to the supine posture. In the upright posture the threshold value will be less than 180 mmHg. The waves are often multi-peaked and prolonged.

Non-specific motility disturbances

In many patients with disordered transit or non-cardiac chest pain, manometry reveals a disturbed motility pattern. When this pattern is not typical of achalasia, diffuse spasm or nutcracker oesophagus, the term 'non-specific motility disturbance' is often applied. Non-specific motility disturbances include abnormalities of amplitude, including isolated waves and failed swallows. Castell has recently questioned this classification and proposed that patients with either non-transmitted or low-amplitude oesophageal contractions should be considered as a distinct manometric category, referred to as 'ineffective motility'[13].

Patients sometimes experience symptoms with normal oesophageal body motility but with sphincter dysfunction. An excessively high sphincter pressure or 'hypertensive sphincter' is usually defined as end-expiratory pressure greater than 30 mmHg above gastric pressure. It is interesting to note that many reports on this condition have documented a high incidence of GOR in these patients[14]. There is some evidence that treatment by dilatation may be helpful in alleviating symptoms in this group.

Secondary motility disorders

Motility disturbances frequently occur secondary to a number of diseases. Systemic sclerosis accounts for a large proportion of patients with secondary motility disorders[15]. When this disorder affects the oesophagus, the amplitude of peristalsis is gradually reduced in the distal oesophagus, and LOS pressure is also reduced, leaving the oesophagus exposed to GOR. There is considerable overlap in clinical features, extra-articular disease manifestations and pathological indices between different connective tissue disorders. Rheumatoid arthritis patients[16] have a 40 per cent incidence of oesophageal dysfunction unrelated to non-steroidal anti-inflammatory (NSAID) drug use.

An association between heart disease and oesophageal disease has long been established, with 50 per cent of patients showing simultaneous symptoms for both. There is evidence of a direct vagal link between the myocardium and the LOS[17]. Stimulation of the myocardial vagal receptors, both pharmacologically (with nicotine) and mechanically, produces a rapid and significant impairment of LOS function. There is also evidence that occlusion of the left circumflex coronary artery produces a significant fall in LOS pressure in the canine model. Frequently, patients with cardiac disease are referred for oesophageal investigations. Cardiac medication should be discontinued but this may not always be possible.

Gallbladder surgery has also been implicated in oesophageal dysfunction. There is evidence[18] of a significant increase in the incidence of GOR and oesophagitis within 3 months of cholecystectomy, which was unrelated to the route of the operation. In this study, 35 per cent of patients had reflux before surgery, increasing to 73 per cent after cholecystectomy. Sphincter pressure and oesophageal body function in the patients studied however, were within the normal range. The probable mechanism of reflux in this group is unknown but TLOSRs and hormonal influences should be considered. Prolonged sphincter manometry may be useful in this group.

Acid infused into the oesophageal lumen induces changes in airway resistance. Atypical symptoms such as chronic cough, chronic aspiration, asthma and laryngitis are now accepted as being associated with reflux disease. In a study[19] of 118 patients with GOR, 63 were found to have respiratory symptoms. The presence of preoperative motility disorder was significantly more common in patients who did not improve after anti-reflux surgery in this study. It has been suggested that respiratory disease interferes with the anti-reflux barrier by influencing the pressure exerted by the right crus of the diaphragm. Clinically, it can be demonstrated that diaphragmatic activity increases proportionally with depth of inspiration and oesophagogastric junction pressure.

Upper oesophageal sphincter

The upper oesophageal sphincter (UOS) is a high-pressure zone between the pharynx and oesophagus, which helps to protect the respiratory tract from aspiration of gastric refluxate and prevents entry of air into the oesophagus during inspiration. Upper sphincter tone increases in response to both GOR and oesophageal acid infusion. During anaesthesia the risk of aspiration is greater as a result of the effect of anaesthetic agents and muscle relaxants, which reduce resting pressure[20].

The UOS is difficult to study. There is considerable axial and radial asymmetry, pressures being higher anterioposteriorly. Pressures are usually much higher than the LOS and the speed of relaxation is considerably faster. The frequency response of perfused catheters is not sufficient to document relaxation with acceptable accuracy. It is also difficult to maintain the position of the catheter in the sphincter during relaxation. For these reasons, perfused catheters are suitable only for measurement of UOS tone. The use of sleeve devices will allow better localization of the sensor in the sphincter, but the frequency response of perfused sleeves is inadequate to measure relaxation accurately. Microtransducer frequency response is better and therefore is recommended for UOS measurement. By surrounding the microtransducer with a column of oil, one can produce a sphincter-measuring device which senses pressure over a 3-cm length. This device is known as a sphinctometer and is potentially useful for UOS monitoring and also for ambulatory sphincter measurements.

Anorectal manometry

Anorectal manometry is widely used but is poorly standardized. The objective is to study the physiological mechanism involved in defecation by monitoring the pressures of the anorectum. This involves the internal and external anal sphincter muscles, which envelop the anal canal and are responsible for the resting and squeeze pressures respectively.

Equipment for anorectal studies is similar to oesophageal equipment in many respects. Most investigators use perfusion or microtransducer catheters. Catheter design is, however, quite different from oesophageal catheters. Sometimes it may be necessary to use several designs of catheter to investigate anorectal problems fully. Resting anal pressure, squeeze pressure, sensation and sphincter length can be measured with a four-channel perfused catheter with sensors 1 cm apart and a rectal balloon attached. Vector volume measurement requires an eight-channel catheter with sensors placed circumferentially at the same level, without a rectal balloon attached. Measurement of compliance requires a single pressure channel, but with a large-capacity rectal balloon attached. A catheter puller is also recommended for vector volume measurement.

Computerized systems for anorectal investigation are widely available. Automatic analysis of anorectal manometry traces is essential for vector volume analysis. However, resting and squeeze pressures can easily be read directly from the trace. Computerization may be helpful in standardization of reports for these investigations.

Manometry is most often requested for patients with faecal incontinence. Digital estimation of anal sphincter, although still used by some, has been shown to be unreliable when compared with objective measurement[21]. Abnormalities may include inadequate resting tone, squeeze pressures or sensation, but some or all of these may be within normal range. A completely normal study will rule out the anorectum as the source of a patient's symptoms. Sensation and compliance may be useful in investigation of neurogenic disorders such as diabetes mellitus[22], multiple sclerosis and nerve injuries[23]. Manometry is also a useful investigation for treatment evaluation – such as in the selection of patients who might benefit from biofeedback retraining, or for pre- and postoperative surgical evaluation.

Manometry is clinically useful in relatively few patients with chronic constipation. Exclusion of Hirschsprung's disease is an important application. Simulated defecation is a useful manoeuvre that may identify inappropriate contraction of the external anal sphincter, also known as anismus. Patients identified with this abnormality may benefit from biofeedback retraining.

The *AGA Technical review*[24] *on anorectal testing techniques* concludes that indications for anorectal manometry are:

- Faecal incontinence: to define functional weakness of one or both sphincter muscles, in which anal endosonography is complementary in demonstrating whether this weakness is caused by anatomical derangement; and to perform and predict responses to biofeedback retraining.
- Pelvic floor dyssynergia: to support findings of other tests and to perform, monitor outcome and possibly predict responses to biofeedback retraining.
- Hirschsprung's disease and anatomical defects of the anal sphincters – vector manometry.

Essential measurements

Maximum resting and squeeze pressures, rectal sensation, sphincter length and inhibitory reflex can be measured using a multi-sensor catheter with a balloon attached. The balloon capacity is usually about 60 ml and is mounted distally on the catheter. It is not necessary to measure inter-balloon pressure for sensation. Pressures in the anal canal can be reported as absolute measurements although usually they are relative to rectal pressure. Care should be taken in introducing the catheter, to ensure that the balloon does not obstruct the pressure sensors. Sometimes it is useful to inflate the balloon rapidly when the catheter has first been inserted in order to avoid this. Generally the length of the catheter inserted is 6–8 cm depending on the catheter design. Rectal pressure should be steady, but often the baseline changes as the catheter is withdrawn. This may be the result of slow-wave activity from the bowel, and if the catheter is withdrawn by 1 or 2 cm the baseline settles down. Stationary withdrawal of the catheter by 1-cm increments will usually detect a high-pressure zone at about 3 cm from the anal verge. With a four-channel catheter at 1-cm spacings, one should continue to withdraw the catheter until the proximal sensor is at the anal verge, the distal sensor is in the rectum or at the lower border of the sphincter, and two sensors are in the anal canal. The presence of an inhibitory reflex, i.e. internal sphincter relaxation in response to rectal distension, excludes a diagnosis of Hirschsprung's disease. However, the absence of the reflex may be the result of other causes such as megarectum where the volume used to inflate the balloon may be inadequate, or the reflex may be absent because of faecal impaction. When the inhibitory reflex appears to be absent, a biopsy should be taken to confirm the diagnosis of Hirschsprung's disease.

Vector manometry

Computerized vector manometry can be helpful in the diagnosis of sphincter injuries by identifying the presence of pressure asymmetry in the anal canal. The computer constructs a three-dimensional anal pressure vector gram from the manometry data, which can be rotated and viewed in several directions by the computer software. The study requires a catheter with four to eight channels, the sensors being at the same level. A catheter puller is attached to the inserted catheter and the pressures are measured during constant withdrawal at a rate of approximately 0.5 cm/s.

It is important to know the orientation of the channels when conducting a pull through. Most manufacturers have a black marking along the length of the catheter. Care should be taken to ensure that this marking stays in one orientation (usually posterior) during the pull through.

Several studies have reported good agreement among vector manometry measurement, ultrasonography and electro-myography (EMG). Perry's[25] vector symmetry index has claimed that this measurement can identify occult sphincter injuries and this has recently been verified by others. Interpretation of vector volume measurements is not yet standardized and the calculation of vector volume in some of the commercially available software packages is not clinically useful.

Compliance

Deferral of call to stool is achieved by the mechanism of rectal compliance. The normal rectum has properties that allow it to maintain a low intraluminal pressure while being filled. The calculation is the difference between the volume at maximum tolerated volume and first sensation, divided by the difference between the pressure generated at maximum tolerated volume and first sensation, expressed in millimetres per millimetre of mercury. The normal rectum is highly compliant and can accept large increases in volume with only a small increase in pressure.

Compliance may be measured using a single pressure channel and a catheter with a large-capacity balloon attached. Intra-balloon pressure is measured for a series of descending volumes that can exceed values of 300 ml of air. The limiting factor is the patient's response. It is useful to document first sensation, urge and maximum tolerated volume. A pressure–volume graph is generated by plotting the balloon volumes from the sensation markers against the adjusted rectal pressures calculated for each of those volumes. The adjusted rectal pressures are calculated from pressures measured in the patient and the pressure exerted by a similar volume when measured outside the patient, thus allowing for the size, shape and the type of material from which the balloon is constructed. Some investigators suggest that water balloon inflation is more reproducible. Compliance is often reported as the slope of the pressure–volume curve expressed as millilitres per millimetre of mercury. Decreased compliance is associated with increased stool frequency and incontinence. Increased compliance is associated with megarectum.

Biliary manometry

Sphincter of Oddi manometry requires an experienced endoscopist and should not be undertaken by a technician. The technique involves the introduction of a multi-sensor pressure catheter into the ampulla of Vater orifice via the biopsy channel of a side-viewing endoscope. The catheter is positioned in the common bile duct. Cannulation is difficult and a guidewire is needed. Care should be taken not to damage pressure sensors if microtransducer catheters are used. Perfused catheters can be used and are available commercially. They usually have three side holes at 2 mm apart. The hydraulic perfusion rate is 0.2 ml/min, which is lower than for oesophageal manometry. A second catheter attached to the outside of the endoscope is also required to measure baseline duodenal pressure. Calibration takes place at atmospheric pressure, outside the patient; perfused sensors should be calibrated at the level of the ampulla of Vater, with the patient supine. Animal studies have demonstrated[26] the influence of the migrating motor complex on gallbladder function.

Practical problems include difficulty in accommodating perfused manometry in an endoscopy suite. If this is a real problem then an ambulatory manometry system may be used. Ambulatory manometry equipment may be used with low-cost perfusion systems, which consist of a pressurized bag connected to pressure transducers with in-built capillaries. The technique is time-consuming and one should consider either having a special session or make sure that the patients for this procedure are at the end of an endoscopy list. Drugs affecting motility should be avoided.

A stationary pull through involves movement from the bile duct into the sphincter of Oddi. Adequate time should be allowed for the pressure tracing to stabilize between catheter movements. Resting pressures are higher than duodenal pressure. Contraction wave frequency is approximately 8/min and the wave pressure can be greater than 100 mmHg. Abnormalities include high frequencies and high amplitudes. It is also possible to measure propagation with this technique, a high incidence of retrograde propagation being deemed to be abnormal.

References

1. Bremner RM, Costantini M, DeMeester TR et al. Normal oesophageal body function: a study using ambulatory oesophageal manometry. Am J Gastroenterol 1998; 93: 183–187
2. Mattox HE, Richter JE, Sinclair JW, Price JE, Case LD. Gastroesophageal pH step-up inaccurately locates border of lower oesophageal sphincter. Dig Dis Sci 1992; 37: 1185–1191
3. McLauchlan G. Oesophageal function testing and antireflux surgery. Br J Surg 1996; 83: 1684–1688
4. Mittal RK, Balaban DH. The oesophagogastric junction. N Engl J Med 1997; 336: 924–932
5. Mattox HE III, Albertson DA, Castell DO, Richter JE. Dysphagia following fundoplication: 'slipped' fundoplication versus achalasia complicated by fundoplication. Am J Gastroenterol 1990; 85: 1468–1472
6. Mugal MM, Bancewicz J, Marples M. Oesophageal manometry and pH recording does not predict the bad results of Nissen fundoplication. Br J Surg 1990; 77: 43–45

7. American Gastroenterological Association. Medical position statement on the clinical use of oesophageal manometry. Gastroenterology 1994; 107: 1865-1884

8. Waring JP, Hunter JG, Oddsdotier M, Wo J, Katz E. The preoperative evaluation of patients considered for laparoscopic antireflux surgery. Am J Gastroenterol 1995; 90: 35-38

9. Hill ADK, Walsh TN, Bolger CM, Byrne PJ, Hennessy TPJ. Randomised controlled trial comparing Nissen fundoplication and the Angelchik prosthesis. Br J Surg 1994; 81: 72-74

10. Stuart RC, Byrne PJ, Lawlor P, O'Sullivan G, Hennessy TPJ. Meal area index: a new technique for quantitative assessment in achalasia by ambulatory manometry. Br J Surg 1992; 79: 1162-1166

11. Richter JE, Castell DO. Diffuse oesophageal spasm: a reappraisal. Ann Intern Med 1984; 20: 242-245

12. Mellow M. Symptomatic diffuse oesophageal spasm: manometric follow-up and response to cholinergic stimulation and cholinesterase inhibition. Gastroenterology 1977; 73: 237-240

13. Leite LP, Johnston BT, Barrett BS, Castell JA, Castell DO. Ineffective oesophageal motility (IEM). Dig Dis Sci 1997; 42: 1859-1865

14. Katada N, Hinder RA, Hinder PR et al. The hypertensive lower oesophageal sphincter. Am J Surg 1996; 172: 439-443

15. Weston S, Thumshirn M, Wiste J, Camilleri M. Clinical and upper gastrointestinal motility features in systemic sclerosis and related disorders. Am J Gastroenterol 1998; 93: 1085-1089

16. Bolger CM, Walsh TN, Gorey TF, Byrne PJ, Hennessy TPJ. Oesophageal function in patients with rheumatoid arthritis. Dis Oesophagus 1993; 6: 47-50

17. Caldwell MTP, Marks P, Byrne PJ, Walsh TN, Hennessy TPJ. Myocardial vagal stimulation impairs lower oesophageal sphincter function. Surgery 1994; 116: 921-924

18. Rothwell JF, Lawlor P, Byrne PJ, Walsh TN, Hennessy TPJ. Cholecystectomy – induced gastroesophageal reflux: is it reduced by the laparoscopic approach? Am J Gastroenterol 1997; 92: 1351-1354

19. Johnson WE, Hagen JA, DeMeester TR. Preoperative oesophageal manometry predicts the response of respiratory symptoms to antireflux surgery. Am J Surg 1996; 131: 489-492

20. McGrath JP, McCaul C, Byrne PJ, Walsh TN, Hennessy TPJ. Upper oesophageal sphincter during general anaesthesia. Br J Surg 1996; 83: 1276-1278

21. Coller JA. Clinical applications of anorectal manometry. Gastroenterol Clinics North Am 1987; 16: 17-33

22. Schiller LR, Santa Ana CA, Schmulen AC. Pathogenesis of faecal incontinence in diabetes mellitus. N Engl J Med 1984; 1307: 1666-1671

23. Caruana BJ, Wald A, Hinds JP. Anorectal sensory and motor function in neurogenic faecal incontinence: comparison between multiple sclerosis and diabetes mellitus. Gastroenterology 1991; 100: 456-470

24. AGA Technical review on anorectal testing techniques. Gastroenterology 1999; 116: 735-760

25. Perry RE, Blatchford GJ, Christensen MA, Thorso AG, Attwood SEA. Manometric diagnosis of anal sphincter injuries. Am J Surg 1009; 159: 112-117

26. Traynor OJ, Byrne PJ, Hennessy TPJ. Effect of vagal denervation on canine gallbladder motility. Br J Surg 1987; 74: 850-854

Chapter 2

Pathophysiological correlations in upper gastrointestinal physiology

SIMON DEXTER

Abnormalities in the function of the gastrointestinal (GI) tract may be secondary to organic disease or occur as a primary failure in the intrinsic control of GI function[1]. Investigations of GI tract function therefore tend to take place after organic disease has been excluded or assessed by radiological or endoscopic examination.

The role of GI physiology in the assessment of upper GI disease may be to identify the cause of symptoms, characterize or quantify the physiological abnormality, direct appropriate treatment and evaluate the response to treatment. Physiological assessment of oesophageal symptoms usually requires at least static pull-through manometry, followed by a 24-hour ambulatory pH study. Ambulatory oesophageal manometry is not widely available but is useful in the assessment of non-cardiac chest pain. Other investigations may include Bilitec assessment of bile reflux and oesophageal scintigraphy.

Gastric physiology is primarily assessed by gastric emptying studies using a radiolabelled meal and scintigraphic evaluation. Other techniques are available to assess gastric emptying, such as ultrasonic gastrography and paracetamol uptake studies. These techniques are useful in the critical care situation when patients are unable to undergo conventional gastric emptying studies. Gastric and pyloroduodenal manometric assessment is possible, but not universally available, and is rarely used in clinical practice. Electrogastrography is also more commonly used as a research tool than a clinical investigation.

In the upper GI tract, GI physiological assessment is most commonly used for the assessment of gastro-oesophageal reflux disease, swallowing difficulties and non-cardiac chest pain. Patients with a variety of dyspeptic symptoms may also come for physiological assessment, as do many with potential complications of reflux but without reflux symptoms. These include patients with asthma and with inflammatory laryngeal pathology. The role of various physiological measurement techniques in each of these circumstances is discussed.

Assessment of oesophageal function

The major indications for oesophageal physiological assessment are reflux symptoms, dysphagia and non-cardiac chest pain.

Gastro-oesophageal reflux disease

Gastro-oesophageal reflux (GOR) affects up to one in five of the adult population. The typical presentation of reflux disease is of heartburn, with or without regurgitation. In most cases it is infrequent and easily managed by symptomatic measures. A significant cohort of people with GOR have more persistent symptoms, or present with complications of reflux such as oesophagitis, oesophageal stricture, Barrett's oesophagus or respiratory disease. Reflux-related respiratory conditions include asthma, persistent cough or even pulmonary fibrosis caused by repeated infection. Patients who develop complications usually require either long-term medical or surgical treatment for their reflux.

The diagnosis of GOR is usually made on the basis of typical symptoms and a beneficial response to antacid or anti-secretory therapy such as proton pump inhibitors. A large proportion of patients, especially older individuals, will have an endoscopy to look for evidence of oesophagitis and exclude other pathology. Endoscopy is not a diagnostic test for reflux disease, although circumstantial evidence of reflux may be gleaned by the presence of oesophagitis or reflux-consistent inflammation from biopsies of a normal-looking oesophagus[2].

More detailed investigation of the oesophagus is reserved for cases where the diagnosis is not clear from symptoms alone or the presentation is atypical, such as respiratory or laryngeal symptoms without obvious heartburn. In addition all patients considering surgical treatment for their reflux should have their oesophageal physiology assessed.

Oesophageal manometry

Acid is the usual cause of symptoms of GOR disease, but the underlying pathology is a disturbance of motility, not of acid overproduction. The predominant causes of reflux disease are failure of the lower oesophageal sphincter (LOS), which allows acid to reflux into the oesophagus, and failure of oesophageal peristalsis, which stops refluxed acid being cleared from the oesophageal lumen. Although manometry may identify an abnormality of the LOS, it cannot be used to diagnose reflux, which requires 24-hour pH monitoring as the gold-standard investigation. Figure 2.1 shows a normal oesophageal manometry recording.

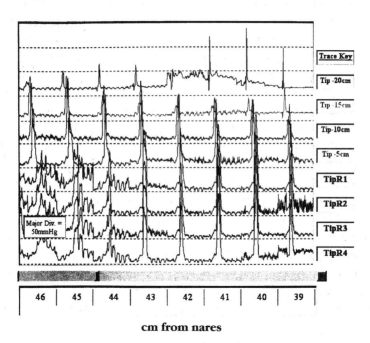

Figure 2.1 Manometry tracing of normal oesophageal function.

The role of oesophageal manometry for presumed reflux disease is to establish the level of the LOS in order to direct placement of a pH catheter, and to quantify any manometric abnormalities of the oesophageal body and LOS.

Typically a patient with GOR has a low basal LOS tone, but relaxation is complete and appropriate following a successful wet swallow. In reflux disease a variety of abnormalities may occur with distal body peristalsis, including failed primary peristalsis, low amplitude peristalsis and simultaneous contractions in the lower oesophagus. Oesophageal spasm may also be precipitated by reflux.

The value of demonstrating these manometric abnormalities is currently limited in terms of their clinical use. Treatment is based on symptoms and complications rather than on the extent of any manometric abnormality. From the surgical standpoint, the most important function of manometry is to demonstrate that the findings are consistent with reflux disease and that the symptoms have not been misdiagnosed. In particular it is important to exclude achalasia of the cardia, because a fundoplication in the presence of untreated achalasia is disastrous.

Other diagnoses that should be excluded are spastic disorders of the oesophagus, which will not respond to anti-reflux surgery unless there is a clear relationship between spasm and reflux episodes. Reflux in the presence of an entirely normal manometric study should also prompt a re-evaluation of symptoms, because reflux is uncommonly a consequence of distal obstruction. If vomiting or large-volume regurgitation and fullness are predominant features, then obstruction should be excluded. The gastric outlet can be evaluated endoscopically, but the proximal small bowel will require a contrast study to exclude an obstructing lesion.

The question of whether anti-reflux surgery should be tailored according to the degree of manometric peristaltic dysfunction has been addressed in the surgical literature. Some surgeons hold the belief that patients with severe oesophageal dysfunction and reflux should have a partial fundal wrap instead of a total 360° fundoplication, to reduce the chance of postoperative dysphagia. There is no evidence to support this contention, and in fact patients with preoperative severe peristaltic dysfunction have been shown to have equally good (or bad) results regardless of whether they receive a partial or total fundal wrap.

Measurement of 24-hour oesophageal pH

The measurement of acidification of the lower oesophagus over a 24-hour period is the most sensitive and specific technique for the demonstration of GOR. Despite its value, limitations to the technique do exist. The most obvious is that only acid reflux is assessed. Reflux will not be demonstrated in the presence of an achlorhydric stomach, whether as a result of continued proton pump inhibitor use or a consequence of atrophic gastritis, which destroys the acid-producing parietal cells of the stomach. Previous surgery on the stomach, including vagotomy, antrectomy or partial gastrectomy, will reduce acid production, but rarely enough to maintain the intragastric pH above 4.0. It is therefore still worth while pursuing oesophageal pH monitoring in these patients if indicated.

Interpretation of the value of a pH study may be complicated because the results are not simply positive or negative, but are represented as a value, which may or may not exceed that seen in most members of a normal population. Reflux is a normal phenomenon that occurs usually at the time of belching, in response to gastric distension. These episodes are short-lived, asymptomatic and rapidly cleared, and are noted manometrically as transient lower oesophageal sphincter relaxations (TLOSRs). When reflux is pathological, reflux events last longer and occur more commonly than in individuals without evidence of reflux disease. The composite DeMeester score, used to assess reflux, simplifies the results of a prolonged pH study into a single value. Six parameters of the study, usually with reference to a pH level of 4.0 (total time < pH 4, upright time < pH 4, supine time < pH 4, number of reflux episodes, number of episodes > 5 minutes and longest duration of a single episode), are each weighted and combined to give a score. The score is compared with the 95th centile of a normal population and is considered abnormal only if it is above the 95th centile.

Although an abnormal preoperative DeMeester score is one of the best predictors of good outcome from anti-reflux surgery, implicit in the score is that it is a simplification. One of the main limitations is that it overlooks the importance of symptom correlation. A small number of patients have DeMeester scores that fall within the normal range, although their frequent short-lived episodes of reflux are clearly the cause of their symptoms when they are scored alongside the pH trace. Patients with so-called acid-sensitive oesophagus usually benefit from anti-reflux measures. Other patients who may experience few symptomatic prolonged reflux episodes in the final score are averaged out by an unimpressive trace for the remaining period. Such patients often report that their symptoms were less than usual on the day of testing, or they avoided the usual stimuli such as eating because of the presence of the pH probe.

By contrast, as reflux is a common phenomenon, patients may have a pathological DeMeester score in the presence of symptoms unrelated to reflux. Caution should be applied to the treatment of reflux for atypical symptoms, unless there is some evidence of symptom correlation. This may not be possible in the case of respiratory or laryngeal disease, where a trial of anti-secretory therapy may prove useful before embarking on anti-reflux surgery. Patients with achalasia may occasionally have acid pH studies as a result of stasis of oesophageal content. In this case the pH gradually falls over time and is cleared when the LOS opens. This pattern contrasts markedly with that of reflux in which the pH drops sharply with each reflux episode.

The use of pH testing after anti-reflux surgery is important. Symptoms after anti-reflux surgery are common, but are unusually the result of recurrent reflux. Nevertheless recurrent reflux does occur in 10–20 per cent of cases, especially in the long term, and may cause symptoms different from those that the patient originally recognized as reflux. Some of these patients have good symptom control after surgery but also have asymptomatic reflux, which can be a cause of ongoing reflux damage.

Radiology

Barium studies are generally not used to diagnose reflux disease because of low sensitivity and a significant false-positive rate. Radiological assessment does have a role in defining anatomy in complex cases such as peptic stricture or para-oesophageal hernia. Rarely the demonstration of definite reflux and the absence of any obvious structural or motility abnormality during contrast radiology may be helpful in decision-making for patients unable to tolerate oesophageal intubation for conventional oesophageal physiology studies.

Treatment of gastro-oesophageal reflux

The treatment of GOR ranges from avoidance of reflux stimuli and mild symptomatic treatment, through continuous medical therapy, to surgery. Medical therapy over and above simple antacids is required in patients with recurrent symptomatic reflux or those with complicated reflux. Oesophagitis is generally treated by a high-dose proton pump inhibitor, stepping down to a maintenance dose after the oesophagitis has healed. In patients with established oesophagitis, withdrawal of acid-suppression therapy results in recurrent oesophagitis in over 70 per cent of patients.

No long-term consequences of extended proton pump inhibitor therapy have been identified in humans, but some health services have not funded long-term treatment. In countries with such health services the rate of surgical treatment is very high. Otherwise, the main indications for surgery are reflux resistant to medical therapy, volume reflux with regurgitation and a desire from the patient to avoid long-term medical therapy.

Surgery addresses the failing LOS complex, rather than just suppressing acid alone, and hence treats the reflux – not just the refluxate.

The major components of the many anti-reflux procedures are to reduce any hiatus hernia and restore a length of oesophagus to the abdomen, narrow the widened hiatus that is commonly observed, and create an anti-reflux mechanism. The most common approach to the latter is to wrap the mobilized fundus of the stomach around the lower oesophagus. The fundal wrap pinches off the oesophagus when the intragastric or intra-abdominal pressure rises, both of which usually precipitate reflux (see Figure 2.2a).

Side effects from surgery are related to the inability to vent the stomach of gas by belching and include postprandial fullness, gas-bloat syndrome, increased flatulence and sometimes diarrhoea. In addition dysphagia often occurs after surgery, although only transiently in the vast majority of patients.

Attempts to avoid such side effects have led to a variety of partial fundoplications being developed[3], in which the fundus is incompletely wrapped either anteriorly or posteriorly around the lower oesophagus (see Figure 2.2b). Each procedure has its advocates, but none appears to avoid side effects and maintain efficacy completely[4].

Investigation of postsurgical symptoms after anti-reflux surgery is an increasing burden on oesophageal physiology, but is often disappointing in its results. Although recurrent reflux is a valuable finding, manometry is often inconclusive in all but the most

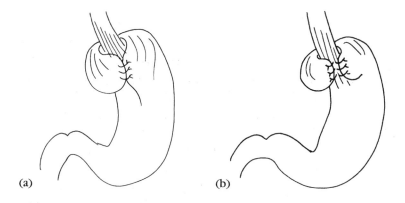

(a)   (b)

Figure 2.2 (a) 360° Nissen fundoplication, (b) Toupet partial posterior (270°) fundoplication.

extreme examples of dysphagia. Despite this, reoperative surgery may be beneficial for both of these complaints.

Assessment of bile reflux

Although acid is the most commonly assessed component of oesophageal refluxate, other injurious components exist. Duodenogastro-oesophageal reflux may damage the oesophagus and is highly prevalent in patients with Barrett's oesophagus, in addition to acid reflux.

Bile can be measured in the oesophagus by the use of a Bilitec probe. The presence of bile is identified by a spectro-photometric technique based on the absorption spectrum of bile. The technique is limited by the need to avoid a range of coloured foodstuffs, which affect the readings, as well as difficulties with solid food, which can block the light source within the probe. Bilitec assessment is rarely used clinically because bile reflux tends to occur at the same time as acid reflux, which is measured more reliably. Acid reflux may not coexist after partial gastrectomy, or during acid-suppression therapy when symptoms or reflux injury persists (see Figure 2.3).

Prokinetic agents may help by improving oesophageal clearance and gastric emptying, but fundoplication will abolish oesophageal bile reflux, because it treats total refluxate. After partial gastrectomy with either a Billroth 1 or Billroth 2 reconstruction, bile gastritis may be the major cause of symptoms, rather than oesophageal reflux. In such cases revision to a roux-en-Y reconstruction is indicated, with or without fundoplication, if oesophageal reflux is present.

Dysphagia

Dysphagia means difficulty swallowing and should be differentiated from problems with eating caused by dry mouth, or problems of volition such as nausea. Mechanical narrowing or obstruction of the oesophagus is characterized initially by dysphagia to solids, but in all cases of dysphagia a contrast swallow or an endoscopy is mandatory before embarking on oesophageal manometry. In addition to the exclusion of mechanical dysphagia, a contrast study may demonstrate features of functional disease such as achalasia or oesophageal spasm (corkscrew oesophagus).

Once a mechanical cause for dysphagia has been excluded, standard oesophageal manometry should be performed. Oesophageal manometry will provide information on the function of the

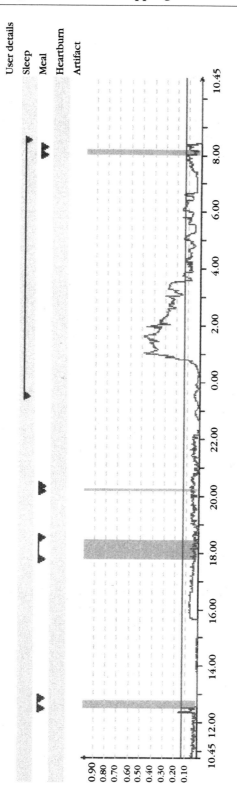

Figure 2.3 Bilitec recording of bile reflux.

upper and lower oesophageal sphincters and that of the resting and peristaltic activity of the oesophageal body.

During a normal swallow pharyngeal contraction sweeps the food bolus through the upper oesophageal sphincter (UOS), or cricopharyngeus. The UOS then contracts behind the food bolus and a peristaltic wave is initiated, which carries the bolus down the oesophagus at a rate of 2–4 cm/s. Preceding the wave of peristalsis is a zone of inhibition of circular muscle contraction (deglutitive inhibition), which accommodates the food bolus and results in relaxation of the LOS as it is reached, allowing the bolus to enter the stomach.

Peristalsis may be primary and initiated in the upper oesophagus, or secondary. Primary peristalsis is that which carries fluid or a food bolus through the oesophagus from the pharynx. Secondary peristalsis can be initiated at any level within the oesophagus by luminal distension, and serves to keep the oesophagus empty.

The majority of functional swallowing difficulties arise in the oropharyngeal phase of swallowing and are usually a feature of underlying neurological disease such as stroke. Swallowing of both liquids and solids is impaired and there are often associated symptoms such as cough or aspiration. In this situation a comprehensive videofluoroscopic evaluation of swallowing is the investigation of choice, because treatment strategies involve anatomically based swallow therapy.

Dysphagia from oesophageal dysfunction can be caused by inadequate or uncoordinated relaxation of either sphincter or by inadequate or disordered peristalsis in the oesophageal body. High amplitude contractions within the oesophageal body (nutcracker oesophagus) can also present with dysphagia as can inflammation resulting from GOR disease.

Upper oesophageal sphincter dysfunction

Failure of relaxation of the UOS (cricopharyngeus) may contribute to dysphagia and is part of the pathophysiology of pharyngeal pouch (Zenker's diverticulum). The treatment of pharyngeal pouch involves fixation or resection of the pouch in combination with division of cricopharyngeus (cricopharyngeal myotomy). Failure to treat the dysfunctional sphincter would lead to inevitable recurrence of the pouch, which is simply a manifestation of the sphincter problem. In such cases, the operation is standard and the decision to operate is based on the symptomatology and the radiological appearances of the pouch, rather than the physiological measurements of the UOS, which do not contribute greatly to management decisions.

Uncommonly, dysphagia is caused by UOS dysfunction in the absence of structural changes and may be suggested by dynamic contrast radiology. Such patients may be candidates for cricopharyngeal myotomy if pharyngeal function is good. Selection for surgery is therefore based on the demonstration of high intrabolus pressure of a bolus in the hypopharynx with failure of cricopharyngeal relaxation. This assessment requires combined fluoroscopic and manometric assessment.

Achalasia of the cardia

Failure of either contractility or deglutitive inhibition will result in failure of bolus progression and will be felt by the patient as dysphagia. Oesophageal manometry is fundamental in determining the specific causes of dysphagia caused by oesophageal dysmotility.

Excessive peristaltic contraction of the oesophagus (nutcracker oesophagus) and diffuse oesophageal spasm are usually associated with pain, although dysphagia may be a feature. More commonly dysphagia occurs because of uncoordinated or hypotensive oesophageal contraction. The most well-defined example of such abnormalities would be achalasia of the cardia (see Figure 2.4).

Achalasia, literally 'failure to relax', is characterized by uncoordinated, non-progressive contractions or aperistalsis within the oesophageal body. In addition the LOS fails to relax on swallowing, and is usually hypertensive at rest.

Achalasia presents with dysphagia as the primary symptom. As the disease progresses the oesophagus dilates proximal to the obstructing LOS, and can harbour large volumes of food, which may be regurgitated or even aspirated if it doesn't pass distally. Patients often lose weight as the symptoms progress. Dysphagia in achalasia is variable and can occur to solids and liquids. Patients may be able to assist oesophageal emptying by employing manoeuvres such as straightening up or lifting their arms.

The underlying mechanism in achalasia is injury to the myenteric plexus. The cause of idiopathic achalasia is unknown, but Chagas' disease, which is a trypanosomal infection most prevalent in South America, closely mimics the oesophageal changes of achalasia. Achalasia may also be mimicked by tumour infiltration around the gastric cardia. It is important therefore to obtain an endoscopic evaluation in all cases and to maintain a high index of suspicion in older patients presenting with apparent achalasia.

Oesophageal manometry is the cornerstone for the diagnosis of achalasia. The pathognomonic features are failure of LOS relaxation and disordered or absent oesophageal contraction, particularly in the distal oesophageal body. The finding of resting LOS hypertension is a common additional feature. Early in the evolution of the disease, some patients may exhibit strong oesophageal contractions on swallowing, although the contractions will yield an isobaric waveform with non-progression. This is known as vigorous achalasia.

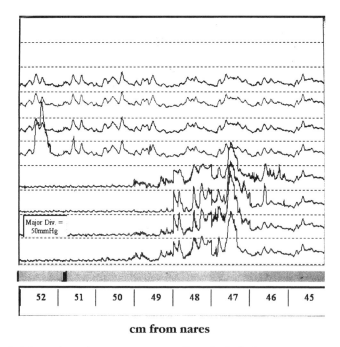

Figure 2.4 Oesophageal manometry recording of achalasia.

Treatment of achalasia

A definite diagnosis of achalasia will prompt treatment, which is usually effective. The main treatment modalities available are surgical cardiomyotomy and balloon dilatation of the LOS. Both procedures are designed to destroy the resting tone of the sphincter. During surgical myotomy the muscle of the oesophageal wall is divided longitudinally across the high-pressure zone of the LOS under direct vision, exposing the underlying oesophageal mucosa. Access to the oesophagus is gained via either the chest or abdomen.

Balloon dilatation is an endoscopic procedure during which a large (3-cm diameter) balloon is placed across the LOS and inflated. Both procedures have their advocates, but surgical myotomy is receiving increasing attention because of the ability to perform the procedure laparoscopically. Moreover, an anti-reflux procedure can be performed at the same time, because reflux is a consequence of an effective cardiomyotomy.

Botulinum toxin can also be injected into the muscle of the LOS as an alternative technique for the treatment of achalasia. It works by inhibiting acetylcholine and thereby paralysing the smooth muscle sphincter. Unfortunately the effect is short-lived, less effective than dilatation, and can make subsequent myotomy more difficult as a result of fibrosis. It is therefore reserved for patients unsuitable for the other techniques.

In addition to making the primary diagnosis, oesophageal manometry has a role in the assessment of achalasia after treatment. Recurrent dysphagia is common after the treatment of achalasia, and may be caused by incomplete destruction of the sphincter, post-treatment scarring or progressive oesophageal body failure. The first two causes result in failure of relaxation of the LOS and may be helped by repeated intervention, whereas recovery of oesophageal body function is impossible.

Successful cardiomyotomy results in GOR in up to 50 per cent of patients. Although unusual before surgery, reflux may contribute to dysphagia in the postoperative phase and should be looked for and treated if symptomatic. There is an argument for routine reflux assessment in view of poor oesophageal clearance caused by aperistalsis and hence the potential for exaggerated complications from reflux disease.

Spastic disorders of the oesophagus

Spastic disorders of the oesophagus tend to present with chest pain, but dysphagia is a common concurrent symptom. The dysphagia is non-specific, affecting solids and liquids, and may be aggravated by stress or other precipitators. The role of oesophageal manometry is discussed below.

Non-specific oesophageal motor disorders

Disturbed oesophageal function that does not fall into specific diagnostic categories on manometry may be grouped under non-specific motor disorders. Non-specific abnormalities may be seen particularly in elderly people, often with symptoms of dysphagia, and may be given the term 'presby-oesophagus'.

Treatment of these conditions is empirical and may be by prokinetics or oesophageal muscle relaxants, depending on the dominant manometric features.

Scleroderma and other secondary motility disturbances

Scleroderma is a vasculitic condition characterized by disorders of the skin, bones and minor blood vessels. Oesophageal abnormalities are common and affect up to 80 per cent of sufferers. Typically patients have dysphagia, with or without reflux symptoms.

Manometry tends to show poor distal oesophageal contraction with LOS hypotension. Upper oesophageal contraction is often better preserved because smooth muscle is affected more than striated muscle. GOR is a common associated feature and should be looked for because some improvement in symptoms can be achieved by its control. The oesophagus may become involved in the neuromyopathies of diabetes mellitus and muscular dystrophy, which usually result in poor peristaltic function and dysphagia.

Treatment of hypotensive motility disturbances is by prokinetic agents. Cisapride was the most effective drug, but it is no longer licensed because of potential cardiac morbidity. Other drugs that may improve motility are metoclopramide and domperidone.

Chest pain

Chest pain is a common symptom with numerous causes. The presence of additional symptoms such as dysphagia may indicate an oesophageal origin. In addition many patients with non-cardiac chest pain will present for oesophageal evaluation after full cardiological assessment has ruled out primary cardiac disease.

Patients with established cardiac disease may suffer non-cardiac chest pain as a consequence of their drugs, many of which relax the LOS, resulting in reflux.

Pain of oesophageal origin may be mucosal or muscular. The character of mucosal pain is readily identifiable as heartburn-like and is aggravated by swallowing, especially hot fluids, alcohol, etc. Muscular pain is less well defined, can be very severe and often penetrates through to the back. Pain may or may not be related directly to eating.

Non-cardiac chest pain originating from the oesophagus occurs in many patients as a result of altered central processing to oesophageal stimuli rather than primary structural abnormalities in the oesophagus. This may account to some extent for the success of centrally acting drugs, such as antidepressants, in some patients.

As with other oesophageal disorders the patient with chest pain will have undergone endoscopy to rule out obvious mucosal abnormality before referral for physiology testing. Contrast studies will also often have been performed and may have demonstrated evidence of a spastic motility disorder. Bolus obstruction resulting from oesophageal stricture can be very painful, but strictures will usually have been diagnosed before physiological evaluation.

Radiology

Contrast radiology may identify a variety of oesophageal abnormalities for which pain may be a presenting feature. However, the specificity of radiological abnormalities such as spasm, tertiary contractions or reflux is relatively low and may not correlate with symptoms.

Oesophageal manometry

Static manometry allows an assessment of swallowing function over several wet swallows, as well as providing a period of observation of resting oesophageal function for the period of the study. In addition, manoeuvres, such as intra-oesophageal balloon inflation, that provoke pain may be reproduced in the laboratory, and symptoms can be correlated with manometric activity.

The two most identifiable spastic oesophageal disorders are diffuse oesophageal spasm and nutcracker oesophagus, both of which can cause oesophageal pain with or without dysphagia. Occasional high-amplitude oesophageal contractions may occur in patients with GOR, and are presumed to be a response to reflux episodes.

Diffuse oesophageal spasm

Diffuse oesophageal spasm is characterized by prolonged, high-pressure, non-peristaltic contractions, usually accompanied by chest pain (see Figure 2.5). Tertiary, non-progressive contractions may be seen endoscopically or represented on barium swallow by the so-called 'corkscrew oesophagus'. An attack of spasm may be precipitated by administration of a cholinesterase inhibitor, such as edropho-nium, in cases of diagnostic difficulty.

Diffuse oesophageal spasm is a characteristic, but uncommon, cause of chest pain. Treatment is by muscle relaxants, such as long-acting nitrates or calcium channel blockers. Patients who fail to respond to drug therapy may be offered balloon dilatation of the oesophageal body or long surgical oesophageal myotomy. Patients with documented GOR experience poorer results after dilatation than patients without reflux.

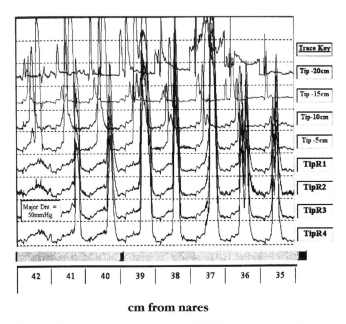

cm from nares

Figure 2.5 Oesophageal manometry tracing of diffuse oesophageal spasm.

Nutcracker oesophagus

High-amplitude peristaltic contraction (> 160 mmHg) is one of the most common manometric abnormalities and is known as nutcracker oesophagus. The relationship between symptoms and manometry may not be clear and hence treatment remains empirical, based on similar principles to diffuse oesophageal spasm (see Figure 2.6).

Ambulatory manometry

Twenty-four-hour ambulatory manometry is available in some laboratories and offers a prolonged assessment of symptom

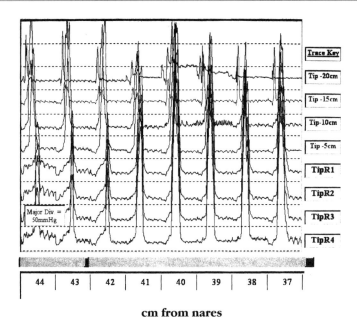

Figure 2.6 Oesophageal manometry tracing of nutcracker oesophagus.

correlation to manometric abnormalities. Indications are relatively few because most symptomatic spastic oesophageal abnormalities can be identified during the examination period of static manometry. However, some patients may be unable to provoke pain in a laboratory setting, and an ambulatory study may pick up the episodes of pain more readily. In addition the number of swallows sampled is up to 100 times greater during an ambulatory test than during a static test.

Study of pH

Gastro-oesophageal reflux is often associated with chest pain, usually heartburn. In patients with documented reflux disease and atypical chest pain, anti-reflux measures improve chest pain in 50–60 per cent of cases, suggesting that spastic oesophageal pain is caused by reflux in some patients. Those patients whose pain clearly correlates with reflux episodes on a pH study can expect improvement in over 90 per cent of cases. It is therefore fundamentally important to establish the presence and extent of acid reflux in these patients and 24-hour pH study should be undertaken as part of their work-up.

Assessment of gastric function

The stomach serves as a compliant, but active, reservoir for food. When food enters the stomach, the proximal stomach relaxes to accommodate the volume and maintains the intragastric pressure at a steady level until the capacity of the stomach is reached. Food is mixed in the distal stomach with gastric juice to form chyme, which is delivered at a controlled rate into the duodenum to undergo digestion. The rate of delivery of chyme to the duodenum is controlled by the nature and volume of food in the stomach, by the intrinsic and extrinsic nerves to the gut and by the interplay of digestive hormones.

Symptoms from functional abnormalities of the stomach often result in abnormal rates of gastric emptying, and gastric emptying studies are the most common investigation of gastric function.

Other investigations of gastric function include manometry of the stomach and pylorus, ultrasonographic gastric motility studies, electrogastrography and studies of gastric compliance using an intragastric balloon (barostat). Few of these additional investigations have found their way into routine clinical practice, however.

Abnormalities of gastric emptying

Symptoms of delayed gastric emptying include vomiting, post-prandial fullness, epigastric pain, nausea, anorexia and heartburn. Accelerated gastric emptying may also give rise to some of these symptoms, but features of dumping may prevail as well. Dumping describes a variety of vasomotor responses such as tachycardia, sweating and fainting. These responses result from fluid shifts related to the osmotic load of chyme in the small bowel, and to swings in blood glucose caused by over-regulation of insulin in response to glucose loads entering the small bowel.

Investigation of gastric emptying is indicated when there is clinical suspicion of abnormal emptying, when empirical treatments for the above symptoms do not appear to work or when symptoms are sufficient to consider surgery (or reoperation). As with all functional investigations, it is important to rule out other pathologies, such as mechanical obstruction, gallstones and ulcer disease, which may produce similar symptoms.

Gastric emptying is usually assessed by scintigraphy following a radiolabelled test meal. Solid and liquid phase emptying are reported separately because these will differ.

Other techniques used to assess gastric emptying include ultrasonic measurements of antral volume after a meal and the paracetamol uptake test. Paracetamol is not absorbed by the stomach and gastric emptying is the rate-limiting step in its absorption. As the stomach empties, paracetamol is absorbed rapidly and completely by the small bowel and appears in the blood, where it can be serially measured.

Delayed gastric emptying

Delayed gastric emptying, or gastroparesis, may be acute or chronic. Acute gastroparesis can occur in response to some drugs (morphine, anticholinergics), is common in critical illness and may occur after non-specific viral infections. Chronic gastric stasis is common in patients with diabetes mellitus, functional dyspepsia, GOR disease and anorexia nervosa. It is also seen as a secondary phenomenon in more generalized myopathies and neurological disorders, and is very common after surgical vagotomy.

Although abnormalities in gastric emptying are common, the relationship of the rate of emptying to clinical symptoms is not clear cut. Delayed gastric emptying is a marker of gastroduodenal motor disturbance and may be a result of poor gastric contraction, poorly organized gastric motility, or high resistance within the duodenum or proximal small bowel. Symptoms may be related to other components of the gastroduodenal disturbance; e.g. abnormal gastric emptying may be found in up to a third of patients with functional dyspepsia, although it correlates poorly with most symptoms except vomiting. In addition many patients, such as those with diabetes, have no symptoms despite markedly abnormal emptying studies.

Severe abnormalities in gastric emptying can cause vomiting of large volumes of undigested food many hours or days after eating, and are a common feature in chronic idiopathic gastroparesis. Weight loss from malnutrition may prevail.

Further evaluation of the specific physiological determinants of delayed gastric emptying is possible, by gastroduodenal manometry and electrogastrography. Current therapeutic options are limited, however, and, provided physical causes such as duodenal obstruction have been ruled out, further investigation is usually unwarranted. This may change in the future as newer treatments such as electrical gastric pacing become established.

Treatments for gastroparesis involve avoidance of precipitators such as high-fat foods and in some cases alcohol. People with diabetes should maintain good glycaemic control because symptoms appear to be worsened by hyperglycaemia. Drugs that promote gastric emptying include the dopamine receptor antagonists metoclopramide and domperidone, and cisapride, which is a serotonin (5HT) receptor agonist. Unfortunately, cisapride has been withdrawn because of cardiac toxicity, and there is no equivalent agent as an alternative. Erythromycin, a macrolide antibiotic, acts as a motilin receptor agonist and is a potent prokinetic agent.

Surgery should be avoided if at all possible because drainage procedures often lack durability of response and result in new functional symptoms. Many patients will end up with repeated surgery, resulting in near total gastrectomy.

Dyspepsia

Dyspepsia may be the result of a variety of upper gastrointestinal causes. Endoscopy is the first-line investigation for dyspeptic symptoms and may reveal a peptic ulcer, gastritis, malignancy or evidence of reflux disease, for example.

Once an identifiable cause of symptoms has been excluded, patients with functional dyspepsia may be referred for physio-logical investigation to categorize them further. Delayed gastric emptying is common in this group of patients, but is not always responsible for symptoms, many of which are no different in similar patients without delayed gastric emptying. Other causes of symptoms may be impaired accommodation of the proximal stomach, or visceral hypersensitivity, both of which can be diagnosed by gastric barostat assessment.

Treatment of functional dyspepsia is often empirical, but detailed physiological evaluation may help guide therapy. Fundal accommodation is induced by sumitriptan, a serotonin $5HT_3$-receptor antagonist, and visceral hypersensitivity may respond to centrally acting anxiolytics or antidepressants.

Postsurgical syndromes

Vagotomy

Operations involving the stomach or the vagus nerves have the potential to alter gastric emptying, producing symptoms such as postprandial fullness, vomiting and the dumping syndrome.

The vagus nerve is responsible for proximal gastric accom-modation and distal gastric motility after eating. Damage to the main trunk of the vagi, either unintentionally or as a planned vagotomy, results in a characteristic pattern of gastric emptying. Liquid emptying is rapid as a result of failure of the proximal stomach to accommodate, whereas solid food emptying is delayed by failure of the antral 'mill' to grind up the meal and deliver it through the pylorus. The addition of a pyloroplasty to truncal vagotomy reduces the resistance across the pylorus and aids solid emptying to some extent.

Highly selective vagotomy preserves the nerves to the antral mill, while dividing the secretory nerves to the acid-producing body of the stomach. Solid gastric emptying is better preserved as a result, compared with truncal vagotomy.

Partial gastrectomy

Gastric resection may be carried out with or without vagotomy, depending on the indication. Whatever the reconstruction, gastric emptying is usually altered. Rapid emptying of semi-solids and liquids may cause dumping, especially after a Billroth 1 or 2 reconstruction. As with post-vagotomy syndromes, solid emptying may be delayed despite rapid emptying of semi-solids and fluids (see Figure 2.7).

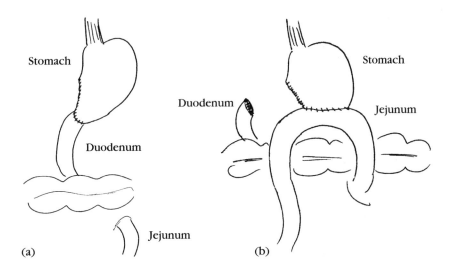

Figure 2.7 Billroth I (a) and Billroth II (b) reconstruction.

Delayed solid emptying is common and is worst in patients with vagotomy. Gastric stasis can occur after roux-en-Y reconstruction as a result of delayed transit through the jejunal loop, as well as from impaired function from the gastric remnant (see Figure 2.8).

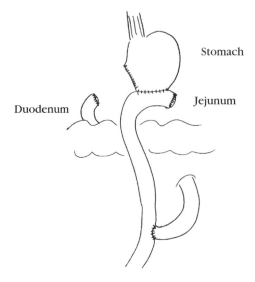

Figure 2.8 Roux-en-y reconstruction.

Most of these syndromes respond to careful dietary advice, concentrating not only on the quality but also on the consistency of the diet. Pro-motility agents may improve solid emptying, but symptoms from rapid semi-solid emptying may be aggravated. Revisional surgery for postsurgical syndromes may be indicated, but results are often not dramatic and may be short-lived. Many patients end up having repeated operations, ultimately resulting in near-total gastrectomy for intractable gastric stasis.

References

1. Phillips SF, Wingate DL (eds). Functional Disorders of the Gut. London: Churchill Livingstone, 1998
2. Kahrilas PJ. Gastroesophageal reflux disease. JAMA 1996; 276: 983–988
3. Lundell L, Abrahammson H, Ruth M, Rydberg L, Lonroth H, Olbe L. Long term results of a prospective randomised comparison of total fundic wrap or semifundoplication for gastro-oesophageal reflux. Br J Surg 1996; 83: 830–835
4. Richter JE. Oesophageal motility disorders. Lancet 2001; 358: 823–828

Chapter 3
Manometry and pH of the upper gastrointestinal tract

LYNNE SMITH

Oesophageal manometry

Measurement of the pressures generated on swallowing provides a quantitative and qualitative assessment of the coordination and motility of the oesophageal body muscle and its sphincters by obtaining pressure profiles. Direct pressure measurement, e.g. an intraluminal microtransducer system, or indirect pressure measurement, e.g. water-perfused catheters connected to external transducers, may be used.

Manometry is the only investigation that enables a precise categorization of primary or secondary oesophageal motility disorders. However, there is conflicting evidence on whether the outcome of the test will influence the type of surgery a patient will undergo, i.e. 'tailoring' of a surgical procedure when taking into account the preoperative motility, although performing the test will help identify patients in whom anti-reflux surgery is inappropriate.

Examples of indications for performing oesophageal manometry[1]

- Dysphagia:
  - evaluation of primary and secondary motility disorders, pharyngeal or upper oesophageal disorders
  - determination of the distance from nose to upper border of lower oesophageal sphincter before placement of pH electrode.
- Preoperative assessment: to exclude primary oesophageal motility disorders before anti-reflux surgery[2].
- Evaluation of patients with 'atypical' chest pain.

Measurement systems

The accuracy of the measuring system is dependent on its ability to reproduce faithfully the rapidly changing pressures generated by the sphincters and the oesophageal lumen during peristalsis. The pressures generated distort a transducer membrane, changing the electrical resistance across it. The resulting changes in electrical signals are modified, amplified, and finally displayed and recorded on a suitably calibrated system.

Direct measurement: intraluminal microtransducer catheters

Although these direct-measurement systems are often called 'solid state', most catheters do not have silicon semi-conductor technology but use miniature strain-gauge transducers. These transducers function in exactly the same way as the standard external blood pressure transducers, e.g. those used in gastro-intestinal tract units or coronary intensive care units (GITUs/CICUs), in that distortion of the diaphragm, by pressure, will result in a change in the signal output that is proportional to this distortion.

The catheters can be made in any configuration, although the spacing of the transducers is usually 5 cm, with a transducer at the very tip (Figure 3.1).

As a result of the asymmetry of the lower oesophageal sphincter (LOS), it is important that the orientation of the transducers along the catheter is such that measurements are made around 360°. Therefore a minimum of three intraluminal transducers with a radial orientation of 120° is necessary. These transducers are very sensitive and careful handling is essential.

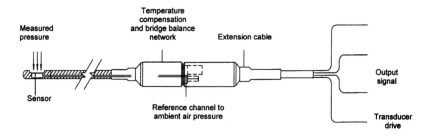

Figure 3.1 Schematic diagram of intraluminal pressure transducer catheter. (Courtesy of Gaeltec.)

Advantages

- Fast response rates
- Can be used for ambulatory recordings
- No water perfusion system required
- Easy to use, sterilize and calibrate.

Disadvantages

- Expensive
- Fragile
- Lifespan depends on how used and cleaned
- Requires cold sterilization methods.

Indirect measurement: perfused system

This system uses an infusion pump to control the rate of water flowing continuously through a multi-lumen catheter to measure pressure indirectly. The pump is usually helium driven (because this is less soluble in water than other gases), and has stainless steel capillary tubing to ensure low compliance and therefore maximum accuracy. The catheter may be of any configuration, depending on the number of pressure transducers available. However, a minimum of three ports, which are radially oriented to allow assessment of the LOS, is required.

Transmission and accurate measurement of a pressure wave, from the opening in the catheter to an external transducer, depends on the compliance of the catheter, the type of perfusion system, the rate of perfusion and the distortion of the membrane on the transducer. Therefore these should be considered before performing a test.

The flow rate of the system should be regularly checked by connecting a syringe to the capillary and measuring the flow over 10 minutes, which should be 0.2–0.6 ml/min. Bubbles of air should be removed from the system and only degassed water used in the pump reservoir. Time should be allowed for the water to perfuse through the capillaries and all the lumina of the catheter before use.

To test the system, occlude one of the perfused lumina on the catheter – the rise rate should be 300 mmHg within 1 second. The lower the compliance of the system, i.e. the stiffer and shorter the catheter and the capillaries on the perfusion system, the more reproducible the pressure changes encountered.

Advantages

- Flexibility in the configuration of the catheter
- Cost-effective
- Disposable catheters and transducers.

Disadvantages

- Stationary studies
- Slow response rate
- Water perfusion system required
- Less suitable for assessment of upper oesophageal sphincter (UOS).

Calibration

The welfare and safety of the patient cannot be over-emphasized when performing any investigation; the system calibration is the most important step to do before patients arrive.

Calibration of all equipment should be carried out before every test. Skipping this step renders the test useless, because the accuracy of the measurements made is the most important aspect of the test. Calibration of intraluminal, or external, transducers is simple, quick and reassuring.

Water-perfused systems are calibrated by applying a column of water that is equivalent to 50 cmH$_2$O to the transducers, or by raising the catheter 50 cm from the predetermined zero level (patient's midaxillary level), and the recording system is adjusted to reflect these pressures accurately.

Intraluminal transducers are calibrated by inserting the catheter into a calibration tube, which has an air seal at one end and a manometer at the other. Usually a positive pressure of 50–100 mmHg (depending on the software/hardware requirements) is applied to the tube and the recording system is adjusted to reflect these pressures accurately (Figure 3.2).

Performing the test

The patient should receive an appointment giving instructions to starve for at least 4 hours before the test. If the patient is undergoing oesophageal manometry only and on the instruction of the referring physician, any medication that will affect the study should be stopped 48 hours before the test. These include:

- Calcium antagonists
- Nitrates

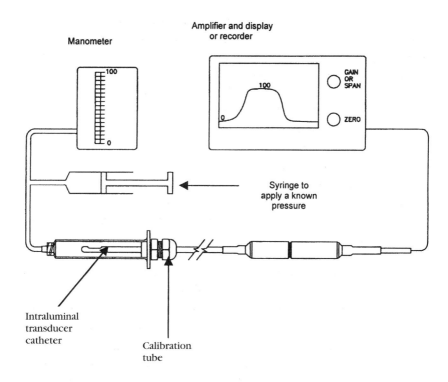

Figure 3.2 Calibration of an intraluminal transducer catheter. (Courtesy of Gaeltec.)

- β Blockers
- Erythromycin
- Prokinetics.

(Please note, when investigating patients who are suspected of having reflux-induced oesophageal motility disorders, that proton pump inhibitors, H_2-receptor antagonists and antacids should also be stopped.)

An informed and written consent should first be obtained from the patient. Compliance with intubation and performance of the test are greatly improved if time is given to explanation of all the procedural details to the patient.

Xylocaine may be applied to the nose and throat, and the catheter lubricated with a water-based gel. The patient will sit with the head flexed during intubation, to reduce the risk of aspiration, and drink water from a straw as the catheter is passed into the stomach. It is important to monitor vital signs of the patient during this period because intubation may induce vasovagal episodes.

When the transducers/recording ports are in the stomach, the patient is allowed an accommodation period. If using a direct measurement system, the patient may remain in a sitting position. If using a water-perfused measurement system, the patient must lie in a supine position with the transducers at midaxillary level. Only when the patient has relaxed and feels that the catheter has been accommodated may the test begin. The patient is requested not to talk during the test and is also discouraged from swallowing unless instructed. This is very difficult for many patients but, with reassurance and time, it should be manageable.

A recording is made while all the recording ports are in the stomach; this is used as a baseline for measuring the resting pressure of the LOS. The catheter is withdrawn in 1-cm increments until the recording channel reaches the distal border of the LOS. At this point the distance from the nose to the distal border of the sphincter is noted. The patient then swallows a 5-ml bolus of water that is at room temperature[3]. Bolus size, consistency, temperature and swallow frequency affect motility, so the test is standardized in this manner to allow accurate assessment of relaxation of the LOS and the resulting response in the oesophageal body. The 'station pull through' is continued until the pressure inversion point is reached; this is the point at which the recording channel has entered the thoracic component of the LOS. The distance from this point to the nose is noted.

The catheter is withdrawn further, and test swallows made, until a drop in pressure occurs as the recording channel enters the oesophagus. This is repeated with all the recording ports until a 360° pressure profile is obtained. The catheter is then withdrawn until at least three transducers are in the oesophageal body. Ten test swallows each of 5 ml room-temperature water are then performed with the catheter fixed in this position. The test swallows are performed every 20–30 seconds, because too-frequent swallows will alter the morphology of the waveforms. If a three-channel catheter is used, it will be necessary to withdraw the catheter and repeat the test in the upper oesophagus (Figure 3.3).

Assessment of the upper oesophageal sphincter

The resting pressure of the UOS is assessed by measuring the mean pressure, over three to four respiratory cycles, in each recording channel. It is important to allow 10 seconds for accommodation, after positioning the catheter, before the measurement is made.

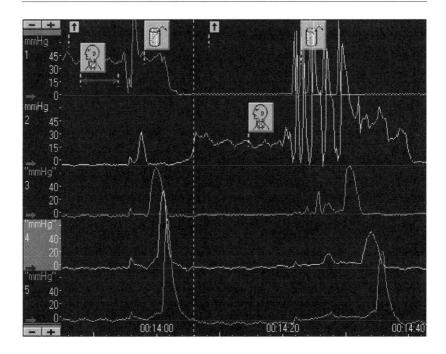

Figure 3.3 Tracing showing the normal response to (a) a single wet swallow (channel 1 = UOS, channels 2, 3, 4 and 5 = in the oesophagus) and (b) multiple rapid swallows and resulting effect on motility. Note only one normotensive peristaltic response.

The coordination of the pharyngeal contraction with the relaxation of the UOS and the initiation of swallow activity high in the oesophagus is an important assessment, particularly in patients who complain of high dysphagia. The catheter is sited with a recording channel in the pharynx, one just proximal to the UOS and one other (or more) in the upper oesophagus. 'Wet' and dry swallows are made. A typical 'M'-shaped waveform is seen in the UOS, with the peak of pharyngeal contraction coinciding with the relaxation of the UOS and a swallow initiated in the upper oesophagus (Figure 3.4).

Analysis

LOS assessment

Figure 3.5 shows that measurements can be made during both the end- and the mid-expiration. When the patient swallows (WS), the sphincter relaxes to allow transmission of the bolus into the

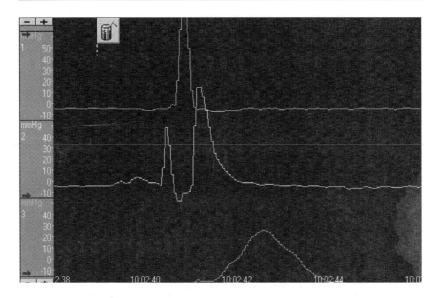

Figure 3.4 Tracing showing the coordination of pharyngeal contraction, UOS relaxation and oesophageal response to a 5-ml water bolus.

stomach. The tracing then rises and settles to the pre-swallow level. Estimation of the resting LOS baseline should be made approximately 10 seconds after relaxation has ended, to allow for cessation of oesophageal movement. When the catheter is further withdrawn to 45 cm, you will note that the respiratory excursions change from positive to negative; this is termed the 'respiratory [or pressure] inversion point' (RIP or PIP) and is the point at which the sphincter enters the chest. The catheter is further withdrawn, in 1-cm increments, until there is a drop in baseline pressure as the catheter enters the oesophagus. A note is made of the length of catheter from the nose to this point (please note that it is 5 cm from this point that the pH catheter will be positioned).

When analysing LOS relaxation, the following should be included in the report:

• The mean end-expiratory LOS pressures from each recording channel.
• The mean mid-expiratory LOS pressures from each recording channel.
• The location and length of the sphincter, i.e. distance from distal to proximal borders of the LOS.

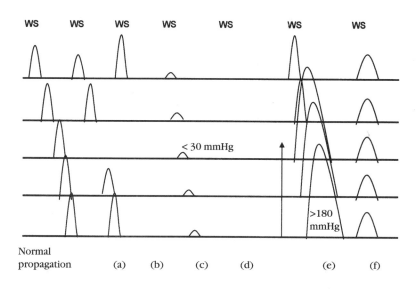

Figure 3.5 Examples of contraction patterns as described above (WS = 5-ml water test swallow).

- The length of the abdominal and thoracic components of the LOS, i.e. the distance from the distal LOS border to the RIP/PIP and the distance from the RIP/PIP to the proximal LOS border.
- The relaxation response, i.e. complete, incomplete or non-relaxing.

The normal LOS:

- Has a mean resting end-expiratory pressure of 10–25 mmHg
- Has a mean resting mid-expiratory pressure of 15–35 mmHg
- Has a predominantly abdominal component
- Should relax completely on each test swallow.

Motility assessment (distal oesophagus)

To assess the 10 test swallows in the oesophageal body, the following should be noted:

- The amplitude of the contraction
- The duration of contraction
- The velocity of propagation
- The morphology of the waveform.

The normal response to 10 swallows of 5 ml water at room temperature is the following:

- The amplitude of contractions is 30–180 mmHg
- The duration of contractions is < 7 s
- The velocity of propagation is 1.7–5.3 cm/s
- The waveforms are single- or double-peaked
- There is propagation of > 80 per cent of test swallows.

Classification of oesophageal contractions

- Interrupted peristalsis (a on Figure 3.5): the swallow is initiated normally but at any point in the oesophagus the peristaltic sequence is interrupted (any 'contraction' of < 10 mmHg is insignificant).
- Non-transmitted episodes (b on Figure 3.5): the swallow sequence is initiated high in the upper oesophagus; however, there is complete failure of the peristaltic sequence.
- Hypomotile oesophagus (c on Figure 3.5): waveforms may be propagated but are of low amplitude (< 30 mmHg).
- Amotile oesophagus (d on Figure 3.5): there is no response to any test swallow.
- Hypercontractile oesophagus (e on Figure 3.5): waveforms may be propagated but are of increased amplitude (> 180 mmHg).
- Incoordinated motility (f on Figure 3.5): waveforms may be of any amplitude but are simultaneous.

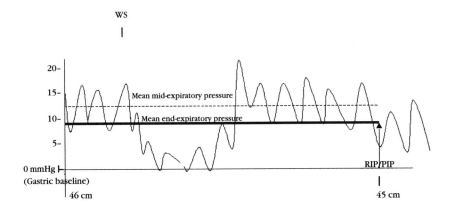

Figure 3.6 Points of measurement and relaxation of the lower oesophageal sphincter.

To simplify the large number of contraction patterns, many are often classified as 'non-specific motility disorders'; the following categorization has been adopted by the Association of Gastrointestinal Physiologists when using a standardized sequence of 10 swallows of 5–10 ml water.

Achalasia (a true primary swallow disorder Figures 3.7a, f)

- Evidence of incomplete LOS relaxation
- Simultaneous distal contractions
- ± Elevated LOS pressure
- ± Elevated oesophageal baseline pressure.

Incoordinated motility (Figures 3.7d, e)

- More than 20 per cent simultaneous contractions
- Intermittent peristalsis
- Repetitive contractions (more than three)
- Prolonged duration (> 6 s)
- Retrograde contractions
- Isolated incomplete LOS relaxation.

*Hypercontracting oesophagus (*Figures 3.7b)

- Hypertensive distal contractions exceeding 180 mmHg
- Increased duration of distal contractions
- Hypertensive LOS.

Hypocontracting oesophagus (inadequate peristalsis Figures 3.7c, g)

- Increased non-transmitted episodes (< 30 mmHg)
- Low-amplitude distal peristalsis
- Hypotensive LOS.

Examples of the causes of secondary motility disorders can include scleroderma, malignancy, neuropathy and mechanical (overtight fundoplication).

Monitoring of pH

The first investigators to use intraluminal pH electrodes to study patients with heartburn found that when patients complained of heartburn it coincided with a fall in oesophageal pH to below 4. Over the years, the test protocol, electrode types and recording systems have been refined, resulting in a 24-hour ambulatory study

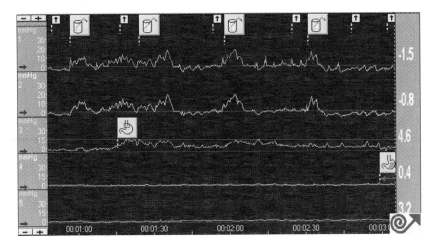

Figure 3.7 Examples of manometric tracings in achalasia, hypercontracting oesophagus, amotile oesophagus (oesophageal involvement in CREST syndrome), incoordinated motility, pseudoachalasia and inadequate peristalsis: (a) Achalasia: recording from a five-channel catheter, sited with distal two recording ports in the stomach. Note the simultaneous multiple-peaked contractions in recording channels 1 and 2 and also the non-relaxing lower oesophageal sphincter in channel 3.

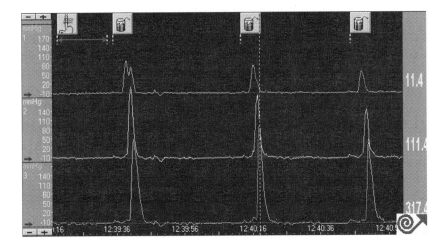

Figure 3.7 (b) Hypercontracting oesophagus: recording from a three-channel catheter with the distal recording port at 3 cm above the lower oesophageal sphincter (LOS). Note waveforms are peristaltic, with normotensive activity in recording channel 1, increased amplitude in channel 2 and hypertensive contractions in recording channel 3. The amplitude of contraction in second test swallow exceeds 317 mmHg. The mean amplitude of contractions in a series of 10 wet swallows exceeds 220 mmHg, although the duration of contraction is within normal limits.

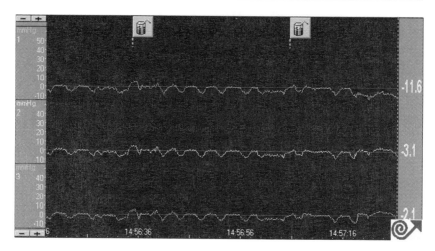

Figure 3.7 (c) Amotile oesophagus: recording from a three-channel catheter with distal recording channel sited 3 cm above proximal border of the LOS. Note nil response to standardized 5-ml, room-temperature-water swallows.

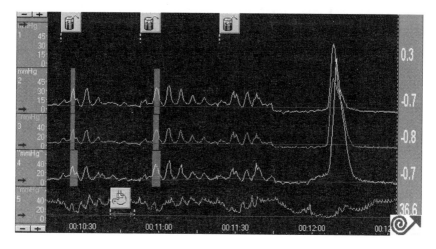

Figure 3.7 (d) Incoordinated motility: recording from a four-channel catheter, sited with distal recording port in the stomach; this example shows low-amplitude and repetitive spastic contractions in response to standardized 5-ml, room-temperature-water swallows in test swallows 1, 2 and 3, with a spontaneous peristaltic hypertensive contraction. The spastic contractions were associated with incomplete LOS relaxation, whereas the peristaltic contraction was associated with normal LOS relaxation. The remainder of the test swallows were normotensive and peristaltic.

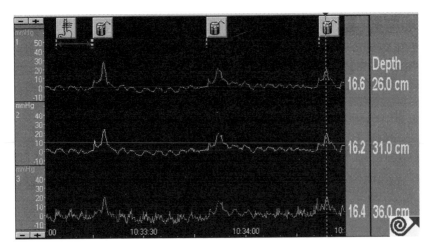

Figure 3.7 (e) Incoordinated motility: recording from a three-channel catheter with distal recording channel sited 3 cm above proximal border of the LOS. Note that all contractions are simultaneous and hypotensive.

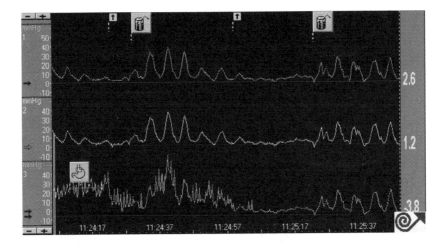

Figure 3.7 (f) Pseudoachalasia: recording from a three-channel catheter, sited with distal recording port in the LOS. This example shows repetitive spastic contractions in response to standardized 5-ml, room-temperature-water swallows with incomplete LOS relaxation. Please note that, in channel 3, as the catheter is withdrawn 1 cm from LOS into the oesophageal body, there is a positive oesophageal baseline pressure, with respect to the predetermined gastric baseline. This tracing mimics exactly the tracing seen in classic achalasia; however, this patient has an extrinsic pancreatic tumour, which is compressing the LOS.

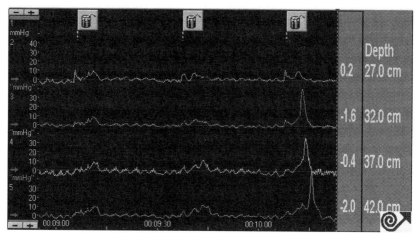

Figure 3.7 (g) Inadequate peristalsis: note very-low-amplitude waveforms in swallows 1 and 2, i.e. < 10 mmHg; these would be classed as 'non-transmitted episodes'. Swallow 3 is normally propagated and normotensive in the distal three channels.

using the fine-bore catheters and miniaturized ambulatory recording systems available today.

Equipment required to perform oesophageal pH metry

- Ambulatory recording equipment
- A pH catheter
- Buffer solutions (typically pH 7 and 1)
- Analysis software
- Personal computer (PC) and printer
- Lubricating gel, anaesthetic spray/gel, adhesive tape, emesis bowls and gloves.

Ambulatory recorders

These are miniaturized, solid-state recorders with a typical memory of between 96 kB and 4 MB. They incorporate an event marker for the patient to press, which will mark the recording when he or she experiences symptoms. The patient will be asked to fill out a diary to make a note of when he or she experiences symptoms, eats a meal and goes to bed. The recorder typically samples the intraluminal oesophageal pH every 1–8 seconds. These data are downloaded on to a computer and analysed with the appropriate analysis software. It is very important to update the software default parameters to comply with current guidelines. It is also essential to ensure that the appropriate changes are made to the software temperature correction factors if you change either catheter type or manufacturer – **always check these details with the manufacturer before use**.

pH catheters

The most commonly used pH electrodes are:

- Glass: the electrode comprises a fine glass bulb, filled with a solution of potassium chloride. A silver/silver chloride wire is in contact with this solution and the pH is determined by measurement of the potential difference between this wire and a reference electrode built into the catheter. These catheters are initially expensive, but are multi-use and therefore, with careful use, can be used up to 20 times. They require cold sterilization after each use.
- Monocrystal antimony (disposable and multi-use): antimony electrodes are usually made from a single piece of antimony, cut from a large crystal. This crystal is connected to a lead with epoxy resin and housed in a PVC tube. The pH is measured by the dissolution rate of the antimony crystal, i.e. the rate at which the surface of the electrode is oxidized by the solution. These electrodes are available as:
  - multi-use, with external reference electrodes, which may be used up to five times for oesophageal recordings and up to three times for gastric measurements; these require cold sterilization;
  - single use, with internal reference electrodes; these **must** be disposed of after use.

Buffer solutions

The pH electrode manufacturers will give guidance on the type of buffer solution to be used for calibration, e.g. **never** use buffers containing phosphates (or oxalate, citrate or tartrate) with antimony electrodes, because complexes which affect the performance of the catheter are formed with the antimony.

System calibration

This is the most important aspect of performing the test. It is a waste of time doing a study **unless** this is carried out, and it must be performed before every recording. If you are unsure of the resulting pH recording, or if there is an unacceptable 'drift' in the overall pH baseline of > 1 pH unit during the 24-hour study, then the catheter should also undergo a check after the pH electrode has been removed from the patient:

- First check the manufacturer's recommended electrode and buffer types.
- Check the software and hardware settings for that electrode type.
- It is very important to make a note of what the correct temperature-correction factors are for every electrode type you use. *The pH is temperature dependent and using the incorrect temperature-correction settings will give you incorrect results. Every electrode type and manufacturer varies.* (As the 'working temperature' is 37°C, a correction factor must be used if calibrating equipment at room temperature, i.e. 25°C; otherwise the buffer solutions should be warmed in a water bath to 37°C and the manufacturer's instructions followed.)

Disposable electrodes (Medtronic)

- Remove the protective sheath around the reference electrode.
- Soak the electrode in pH 7 buffer solution for approximately 10 minutes.
- Put a new 9.0-V battery into the pH recorder.
- Check the correction factors and set-up of the ambulatory pH recorder.
- 'Zero' the recorder, i.e. erase the last patient recording.
- Calibrate in pH 7 and then in pH 1 (some manufacturers recommend pH 4 as the 'low' pH calibration).
- Clean and dry the electrode and re-immerse in pH 7. Set recorder to 'record' and check that this reads **pH 6.0** at 25°C in pH 7 buffer.
- Check that the software reflects the electrode type and the appropriate correction factors; e.g. when using a Medtronic disposable electrode, 'low' = 0.7, 'high' = 1.0. The software will then automatically adjust the patient's recording to reflect the type of calibration method used, i.e. pH 6 calibrated at 25°C = pH 7 at 37°C.

Semi-disposable electrodes (Medtronic)

- Place both the recording and reference electrode in a pH 7 buffer solution for approximately 10 minutes.
- Put a new 9.0-V battery into the pH recorder.
- Check the calibration factors and set-up of the ambulatory pH

recorder (i.e. choose semi-disposable antimony and set the calibration at 'low' pH = 0.8 and 'high' pH = 6.7).

- 'Zero' the recorder, i.e. erase the last patient recording.
- Calibrate in pH 7 and then in pH 1.
- Clean and dry the electrode and re-immerse in pH 7. Set recorder to 'record' and check this reads **pH 6.7** at 25°C in pH 7 buffer.
- Check that the software reflects the electrode type and the appropriate temperature-correction factors, i.e. 'low' = 0.2, 'high' = 0.3. The software will then automatically adjust the patient's recording to reflect the type of calibration method used, i.e. pH 6.7 calibrated at 25°C = pH 7 at 37°C.

If in doubt, contact the equipment/electrode manufacturer.

Indications for test

- Investigation of endoscopy-negative patients with symptoms of gastro-oesophageal reflux
- Patients with atypical symptoms, e.g. non-cardiac chest pain, atypical dental erosion, late-onset asthma, persistent cough
- Pre- and postoperative anti-reflux procedure assessment
- Evaluation of medical therapy.

Contraindications for test

- Nasopharyngeal/upper oesophageal obstruction
- Severe uncontrolled coagulopathy
- Severe maxillofacial trauma and/or basilar skull fracture
- Bullous disorders of the oesophageal mucosa
- Unstable angina
- Poor tolerance of vagal stimulation
- Recent gastric surgery
- Oesophageal tumours or ulcers
- Oesophageal varices
- Poor patient compliance.

Possible complications of intubation and extubation

- Nasal or pharyngeal trauma, haemorrhage
- Laryngeal trauma
- Nasotracheal intubation
- Oesophageal trauma/perforation
- Vomiting

- Vasovagal syndrome
- Bronchospasm
- Could trigger trigeminal neuralgia
- Introduction/transmission of infection
- Mucosal damage
- Entrapment of catheter.

Protocol for test

- Appointments sent to patients should include test information, when to fast from and, importantly, instructions on what medication to stop and when to stop it. This should be confirmed with the referring consultant:
  - drugs to stop 7 days before the tests: proton pump inhibitors
  - drugs to stop 48 hours before the tests: H_2-receptor antagonists, prokinetics, calcium antagonists, β blockers, nitrates, erythromycin
  - drugs to stop the day of tests: antacids, alginates, glyceryl trinitrate spray.
- The patient should have undergone oesophageal manometry before the pH test, during which the distance from the nose to the upper border of the LOS will be measured. Assessment of motility is important because many patients with primary motility disorders have typical reflux symptoms and, not infrequently, normal barium and endoscopic findings.
- Following informed and written consent (this may be given before performing oesophageal manometry) and application of local anaesthetic, the patient should sit with the head flexed, which encourages closure of the trachea. The catheter is passed into the back of the nose and the patient is then requested to sip water through a straw (keeping the head flexed). Never push the catheter – always aid the catheter movement forward as the patient swallows – otherwise kinking/curling and trauma can occur. If the patient coughs excessively, the pH catheter may have passed into the trachea or the patient may have inhaled water. Pull the catheter back and allow time for the patient to recover his or her composure – never rush this. Repeat until the catheter passes into the stomach, i.e. 10 cm longer than the previously determined length from the nose to the proximal border of the LOS.
- If using an electrode with an external reference electrode, apply electrolyte gel to the cup of the electrode (this **must** be of a

similar electrolyte composition to the buffer solution used; if unsure ask the equipment manufacturer). Apply an adhesive ring and attach to clean, dry skin.

- Connect the ambulatory pH recorder and confirm that the catheter is in the stomach, i.e. the pH should be approximately 1–2.
- Withdraw the catheter until it is positioned 5 cm above the proximal border of the LOS.
- Secure catheter at the nose and on face/neck, to ensure that accidental withdrawal of the catheter does not occur.
- Position the electrode lead under the patient's clothing.
- Give the patient instructions on how and when to press event button(s) on the recorder and also what information to include in a diary over the next 24 hours.
- Fizzy pop, fruit juices, squash and alcohol are forbidden; otherwise, the patient carries on with his or her usual routine (and should be encouraged to do so) as long as he or she writes down relevant information in the diary.
- Baths and showers are forbidden because the equipment is not usually waterproof.
- The patient should be asked **not** to swallow chewing gum because this sticks to the catheter!
- Explain how to remove the catheter in the event of vomiting (should the electrode be expelled through the mouth). This is a possibility and these instructions will prevent undue anxiety should it occur.
- Give the patient an appointment for the following day for removal of the catheter and return of equipment.

Analysis of pH recordings

Figure 3.8 illustrates the occurrence and duration of an acid reflux event, i.e. the duration of a drop in pH below 4.

Acid reflux event

- A significant reflux event is a drop in pH below 4 for longer than 5 minutes.
- The end of a reflux event occurs when the pH reaches 5.
- In a normal individual, the pH should **not** drop below 4 for greater than 4.5 per cent of the 24-hour period.
- The symptom index is the proportion of reflux episodes corresponding to a patient's symptom event:

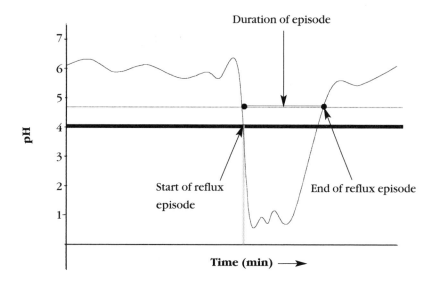

Figure 3.8 The occurrence and duration of an acid reflux event, i.e. the duration of a drop in pH below 4.

$$\frac{(\text{Number of patient symptoms when pH} < 4) \quad \times \quad 100}{\text{Total number of symptoms}}$$

- A 'normal' study period with good symptom correlation (> 50 per cent) is a significant test.

References

1. British Society of Gastroenterology. Guidelines for Oesophageal Manometry and pH Monitoring. London: British Society of Gastroenterology, 1996
   Evans DF, Buckton GK (eds). Clinical Measurement in Gastroenterology. Oxford: Blackwell Science, 1997
2. Mughal MM, Bancewicz J, Marples M. Oesophageal manometry and pH recording does not predict the bad results of Nissen fundoplication. Br J Surg 1990; 77: 43–45
   Stendall C (ed.). Practical Guide to Gastrointestinal Function Testing. Oxford: Blackwell Science, 1997
3. Winship DH, Viegas de Andrade SR, Zboralske FF. Influence of bolus temperature on human esophageal motor function. J Clin Invest 1970; 49: 243–250

Chapter 4
Breath testing and its interpretation

JP Vasani and Herr Hsin Tsai

Breath tests have been valuable tools in the diagnosis of various gastrointestinal diseases for almost three decades. They have assumed even greater importance in the last 10 years, after the discovery of *Helicobacter pylori* and the recognition of lactose intolerance and bacterial overgrowth as important causes of diarrhoea in patients. However, despite their long history they remain, in our view, underused, mainly as a result of unavailability and unfamiliarity, especially in district hospitals in the UK. Here we review their physiological basis, techniques and current clinical applications.

History

Breath tests were introduced in the 1970s initially for diagnosis of lactose malabsorption. Newcomer et al. in 1975 compared hydrogen breath testing with carbon-dioxide-labelled lactose and blood glucose measurements[1]. Subsequent studies[2, 3] confirmed its reliability and often superiority over other tests, and the breath test is now the initial test of choice for diagnosis of lactose malabsorption. Based on the same principles, it was soon applied to malabsorption of other sugars such as fructose[4], maltose[5] and sucrose[6].

In the late 1970s hydrogen breath analysis was reported also to be useful as a diagnostic test for intestinal bacterial overgrowth by Metz et al.[7], who used glucose as a substrate, and subsequently by Rhodes et al.[8] using lactulose. Diggory et al.[9] showed that breath analysis could be used to measure orocaecal transit time in normal individuals and that this could be reliably reproduced.

The interaction between hydrogen and methane (CH_4) production was realized in the 1980s[10, 11] and this led to the incorporation of CH_4 analysis in order to improve the sensitivity of breath tests.

The discovery of *H. pylori* as the predominant cause of peptic ulcers in humans in the early 1980s[12] led to the development of several diagnostic tests. The urea breath tests were soon described for this and are now part of routine clinical practice. More recently, breath tests have been reported in the assessment of liver and pancreatic function, although these have not yet gained widespread acceptance.

Physiological aspects

Although breath tests are used currently for a number of clinical applications the basic physiological principle underlying all breath tests is the same. A substrate, usually a sugar, is introduced into the gastrointestinal (GI) tract. This is metabolized by bacteria or an enzyme and a gas is produced, which is excreted via the lungs. This gas is analysed either quantitatively or qualitatively, and interpreted in the appropriate context. Besides the diagnosis of *H. pylori*, infection breath tests are most commonly used in the diagnosis of carbohydrate malabsorption and bacterial overgrowth syndromes. An understanding of normal carbohydrate digestion, gut bacterial flora and gas production in the normal gut is therefore essential, and is reviewed briefly:

- Normal carbohydrate digestion and absorption
- Role of colonic bacteria
- Normal gas production in the GI tract – role of methane.

Normal carbohydrate digestion and absorption[13]

Chemically, carbohydrates can be subdivided into mono-, di-, oligo- or polysaccharides, depending on the length of the constituent molecular chains. The monosaccharides include simple sugars such as glucose, fructose, galactose, mannose (hexoses or six-carbon molecules) and D-xylose (pentoses or five-carbon molecules). The disaccharides are formed by combining two individual monosaccharides and include sugars such as lactose (glucose + galactose), sucrose (glucose + fructose) and maltose (glucose + glucose). Lactulose and lactitol are examples of oligosaccharides that are not normally digested by gut enzymes. Polysaccharides are complex and large carbohydrates that have to be digested to simpler monosaccharides in order to be absorbed. The main dietary polysaccharide includes starch, which is a long chain of glucose molecules existing as either amylose or amylopectin.

In the Western diet about 45 per cent of the total energy requirement is provided by carbohydrate, which exists in two forms: an available or digestible form and an unavailable or indigestible form. The two main sources of digestible carbohydrate are starch, derived from cereals or plants, and sugars, derived from milk (lactose), fruits (fructose), and cane or beet sources (sucrose, table sugar). Most of the unavailable or indigestible carbohydrates are made up of non-starch polysaccharides, including the so-called dietary fibre, which consists of cellulose and hemicellulose. Pectins, gums and alginates are other unavailable carbohydrates.

In the human gut, digestion of carbohydrate involves an initial intraluminal phase in which starch is hydrolysed chiefly by pancreatic amylase, producing short oligosaccharides, maltotriose, maltose and dextrins. These, together with the major dietary disaccharides (sucrose and lactose), are hydrolysed by specific brush-border enzymes, including lactase, maltase and sucrase-isomaltase present maximally in the duodenal and jejunal villi. This combination serves to liberate glucose monomers that are efficiently absorbed by saturable, carrier-mediated transport systems also located in the brush-border membranes of enterocytes.

It is not difficult therefore to envisage that carbohydrate maldigestion and malabsorption could result from a breakdown of any of the individual steps, resulting in undigested substrate being transported to the colon and so causing clinical problems.

Role of intestinal bacteria

In adults, gastric acidity ensures that the stomach and proximal small intestine contain very small numbers of bacteria that are clinically insignificant in health. The relatively high pH and the negative redox potential in the ileum allows concentrations of micro-organisms to increase to levels of 10^3–10^5 organisms per gram of contents. These include members of the Enterobacteriaceae – coliforms and anaerobes. Across the ileocaecal valve the total number of bacteria increases up to one-million-fold and is highest in the colon. In health the colonic flora are dominated by fastidious anaerobes such as *Bacteroides* species, lactobacilli and *Clostridium* species.

In health colonic bacteria metabolize several substrates[14-17] including lipids, proteins, carbohydrates, bile acids and drugs. They hydrolyse glycerides and synthesize lipids from simpler organic compounds such as acetate. Proteins and urea are degraded to produce ammonia, which is implicated in the pathogenesis of hepatic encephalopathy. Colonic bacterial disaccharidases split unabsorbed dietary sugars and ferment them to produce short-chain fatty acids. These help to conserve calories and are also important for the normal integrity of the colonic mucosa. They help to metabolize drugs such as sulphasalazine and balsalazide into their active metabolites, and may be important in the pathogenesis of inflammatory bowel disease and colon cancer.

Normal gas production and elimination in the bowel

Normal bowel gas comprises five constituents: N_2, O_2, CO_2, H_2 and CH_4. There are three main sources of these gases: swallowed air, intraluminal production and diffusion from the blood. Likewise there are three main routes of elimination: eructation, diffusion into the bloodstream and subsequent excretion in the breath, and finally as flatus. Bacterial metabolism also plays a role in elimination of H_2 as discussed below.

Nitrogen and oxygen are derived mostly from swallowed air, and are eructated. Variable amounts diffuse into the bloodstream and are excreted in the breath, whereas they are present only in small quantities in flatus.

The main source of CO_2 in the upper bowel is from the interaction of hydrogen and bicarbonate. In the colon, on the other hand, CO_2 mainly comes from bacterial fermentation, making up 50–60 per cent of flatus. From the proximal bowel variable amounts of CO_2 diffuse into the blood and from there into the breath.

In the human gut the sole source of H_2 is from bacterial metabolism. In the absence of bacterial overgrowth in the small bowel, H_2-producing bacteria are present only in the colon and depend mainly on exogenous substrates to generate H_2. These substrates include carbohydrates and proteins, which may be maldigested and/or malabsorbed, or normally present in foods such as beans, wheat, oats, certain sweeteners and fibres. Hydrogen thus produced is used by bacteria for further reactions, including the generation of methane, or is excreted by way of the rectum or the lungs.

Like H_2, CH_4 is produced in humans solely by bacteria. About one-third of adults have a large number of methanogenic bacteria and therefore excrete appreciable amounts of CH_4 in the flatus or breath. The interaction between H_2 and CH_4 production is complex and not well understood. In some individuals methanogenic bacteria are present in significant numbers and able to convert H_2 into CH_4. Both H_2 and CH_4, when present in the gut, diffuse rapidly into the blood by virtue of their partial pressures and are excreted almost immediately by the lungs. Depending on the relative numbers of H_2- or methane-producing bacteria, therefore, when a disaccharide is metabolized, sometimes H_2 alone is produced, sometimes both H_2 and CH_4 are produced and sometimes only CH_4 will appear in the breath. The appearance of either or both in the breath is indicative of bacterial activity.

Given that carbohydrates that reach the colon can be metabolized by bacteria into H_2 and/or CH_4, it is common for these to be detected in breath analysis. The fasting H_2 levels are, however, usually less than 10 p.p.m. (parts per million), but these can vary greatly[18]. Foods such as beans can increase fasting breath H_2 levels, as can sleep, during which intestinal motility is reduced, allowing H_2 levels to accumulate[19].

Clinical applications

In the gastroenterology literature, breath tests have been reported to be of use in the following:

- Lactose intolerance
- Intestinal bacterial overgrowth
- Intestinal transit time
- Diagnosis of *H. pylori* infection
- Other less common uses:
    - malabsorption of other sugars (glucose, fructose, maltose)
    - bile salt malabsorption
    - to test for pancreatic exocrine function
    - quantitative liver function.

Lactose intolerance

Principle

The enzyme lactase in the jejunum normally hydrolyses lactose in milk to glucose and galactose, which are readily absorbed. The levels of lactase in the small intestine are genetically determined in an autosomal dominant fashion and begin to decline after 3–5 years of age. The ability to digest lactose therefore depends on the levels persisting into adulthood. Lactase deficiency results in lactose malabsorption and – if associated with diarrhoea, abdominal cramps and flatulence – is termed 'lactose intolerance'.

The absence of lactase and the resultant maldigestion of lactose lead to increased delivery of undigested lactose to the colon, where it is fermented by bacteria producing hydrogen and methane, which can be detected in breath. This forms the basis for the hydrogen breath test, which is the test used most commonly to diagnose lactose intolerance.

The other methods used to diagnose lactose intolerance include a trial of a lactose-free diet, blood glucose measurements after an oral lactose load, and estimation of lactase activity in vitro in histology specimens of the jejunum obtained endoscopically. The H_2 breath test is, however, simple, non-invasive and more reliable than the blood test[20, 21], and is therefore the initial diagnostic test of choice.

Test protocol

Patients are asked to avoid foods such as beans, bran or other high-fibre cereals on the day before the test. Antibiotics should not have been used 2 weeks before the test. After an overnight fast, two baseline breath samples are obtained and analysed for H_2 and, if appropriate, methane. The fasting values should usually be less than 10 p.p.m. Then 25 g lactose (1 g/kg in children) is given orally, dissolved in water. Further samples of breath are then collected at 30- to 60-minute intervals for up to 3 hours. Many stop the test if interval samples show a rise in H_2 of more than 20 p.p.m.

Interpretation (Figure 4.1)

If lactose digestion is normal, lactose is completely hydrolysed by lactase and there is no significant change in the breath H_2 levels during the test. If the patient lacks the enzyme lactase and is consequently unable to digest lactose, the breath H_2 rises by 20 p.p.m. between 1 and 2 hours after the ingestion of lactose, reflecting the time taken for it to reach the colon.

Limitations

Although the test has a high overall sensitivity and specificity, there are occasionally problems. High fasting H_2 values may occur in

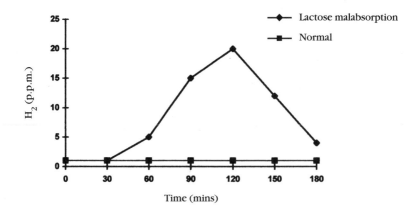

Figure 4.1 Typical lactose H_2 breath test findings in normal and lactose-intolerant individuals.

patients who have not fasted adequately or have eaten high-fibre or slowly digested foods on the previous day, and also in the presence of bacterial overgrowth in the small intestine.

In about 5–18 per cent of patients with lactose intolerance, false-negative tests occur, i.e. there is no rise in breath H_2 despite lactose maldigestion[22, 23]. This can be the result of various causes, including the use of antibiotics, which can sterilize the colon[24], use of laxatives and enemas, or conditions that increase colonic transit[25]. Five to ten per cent of patients do not produce H_2, as a result of the presence of flora that either are incapable of generating H_2 or produce methane instead[26]. If lactose intolerance is strongly suspected clinically, this can be overcome by using a methane analyser simultaneously or using an alternative substrate such as lactulose[27].

False-positive tests, i.e. high H_2 values despite normal lactose digestion, are rare and are usually the result of improper patient preparation[28]. Smoking by the patient or by anyone else in the test area may also result in a false-positive test.

Intestinal bacterial overgrowth

Principle

As mentioned earlier, the normal small intestine is free of bacteria. Several defence mechanisms are responsible for this, including the cleansing effect of normal peristalsis, gastric acidity, the presence of an intact ileocaecal valve, secretory immunoglobulins and pancreatic/biliary secretions, which have some bacteriostatic properties.

Conditions that affect intestinal motility, including scleroderma, diabetes, hypothyroidism[29] and surgical anastomoses, help cause stagnation of intestinal contents, promoting bacterial overgrowth. This may result in symptoms of abdominal discomfort, bloating and diarrhoea[30]. Bacteria also interfere with the absorption of fats, vitamins and sugars, leading to the so-called bacterial overgrowth syndrome.

When these bacteria are exposed to substrates administered orally, the resultant metabolites are excreted in breath, where they can be measured. This is the principle behind breath tests used to diagnose bacterial overgrowth.

Four substrates have so far been reported as being used in breath tests to diagnose bacterial overgrowth. The ^{14}C-labelled bile acid, choleglycine, was the first described[31]. However, interpretation can be difficult and, in view of a high false-negative rate of 30–40 per cent, it is hardly used anymore. The other ^{14}C-labelled test is the 1-gram xylose breath test, in which elevated levels of $^{14}CO_2$ appear in the breath in 85 per cent of patients within 60 min[32]. This test also involves a small dose of radioactivity.

The glucose and lactulose H_2 breath tests are used most commonly and measure H_2 released during bacterial fermentation of glucose or lactulose. Glucose is normally absorbed in the small intestine before it gets to the colon. Lactulose, on the other hand, is not hydrolysed until it reaches the colon. Therefore if a response appears soon after glucose or lactulose ingestion it is suggestive of bacterial overgrowth.

Test protocol

Patients are asked to avoid foods such as beans, bran or other high-fibre cereals on the day before the test. Antibiotics should not have been used 2 weeks before the test. After an overnight fast two baseline breath samples are obtained and analysed for H_2 and, if appropriate, methane. The fasting values should usually be less than 10 p.p.m.

The patient is then given either glucose 70–100 g or lactulose 10 g dissolved in 200–250 ml water. Breath samples are collected every 20 minutes for at least 2 hours after glucose and for 3 hours after lactulose.

Interpretation (Figure 4.2)

If glucose is used, an increase of at least 12 p.p.m. over baseline values indicates bacterial overgrowth. In the absence of bacteria, glucose will be absorbed entirely and there will be no response. If bacteria are present in the proximal small intestine, H_2 appears in the breath within 20–60 min.

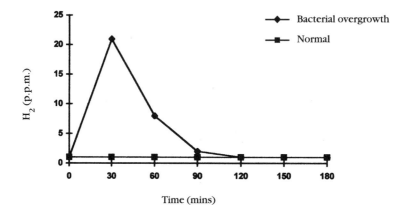

Figure 4.2 Typical glucose H_2 breath test findings in normal and intestinal bacterial overgrowth.

If lactulose is used as the test substrate then bacterial overgrowth classically generates a bimodal peak in breath H_2 (Figure 4.3). The first peak occurs early, usually within 20 min, followed by a much larger peak resulting from normal colonic bacteria. This second peak occurs after an hour and is sustained.

The sensitivity and specificity of the H_2 breath tests, if well conducted, approach 90 per cent in some studies, although this is disputed by some[33-35]. The specificity can be increased even further by combining the observation of an elevated fasting breath H_2 level (> 20 p.p.m.) with a positive H_2 response to the challenge dose (> 12 p.p.m.)[36-38]. The added measurement of methane may reduce the false negatives sometimes seen in non-H_2 producers. One advantage of using lactulose is that it is carried further down the jejunum, thereby increasing the sensitivity of the test in patients with bacterial overgrowth more distally in the small bowel.

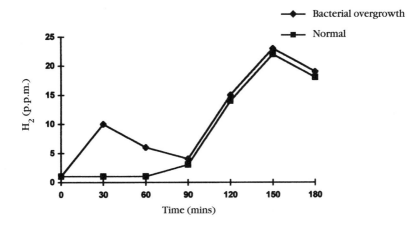

Figure 4.3 Typical lactulose H_2 breath test findings in normal and intestinal bacterial overgrowth.

Intestinal transit time

Principle

As noted earlier, lactulose cannot be digested by humans and therefore it passes to the colon unchanged where it is fermented by bacteria to produce H_2 and/or CH_4, which is excreted in the breath. The time taken for H_2 to appear in the breath therefore gives an indirect measure of small intestinal or, more correctly, orocaecal transit.

Measurement of the orocaecal transit time (OCTT) is used mainly in evaluating patients with constipation. The OCTT is affected by several factors as discussed below.

Test protocol

As with other breath tests, the patient avoids high-fibre foods and other carbohydrates such as beans, and fasts overnight for 12 hours. Antibiotics should not have been used for at least 2 weeks before the test.

A baseline breath sample is collected and H_2 levels are analysed. The patient is then given 10 g lactulose, and breath samples are collected after 30 min at 10- to 20-min intervals. The test is stopped after 5 hours or when there is a rise in H_2 of at least 3 p.p.m. for three successive periods. The time for the first sustained increase in breath H_2 is taken as the OCTT. If there is an early increase (< 30 min) the test should be extended to 3 hours to ensure that the early rise is not caused by intestinal bacterial overgrowth.

Interpretation

The normal OCTT is usually about 75 min with a wide normal range from about 60 to 110 min.[39-41] Several factors affect the OCTT. Lactulose itself can increase intestinal motility, as a result of its osmotic effect, and therefore shorten the OCTT. It is important to use a small dose, with 10-15 g being the usual maximum recommended[42, 43]. Diseases such as cystic fibrosis[44], Crohn's disease[45] and obesity[46] prolong the OCTT, as does smoking[47]. The OCTT is also affected by psychological mood[48], anorexia nervosa and pregnancy[49, 50]. Intestinal transit is shortened by thyroid diseases[51]. In non-H_2-producers, there will be no rise in breath H_2 even after 5 hours. Breath CH_4 can be used in these patients. It is important also to recognize the difference between a rise in breath H_2 caused by bacterial overgrowth and the rise used to measure the OCTT. In the presence of bacterial overgrowth there is usually an early peak, followed by a later, more sustained one.

Diagnosis of *H. pylori* infection

Principle

Helicobacter pylori has now been accepted as the most important cause of peptic ulcers. It causes about 90-95 per cent of duodenal ulcers and about 80-85 per cent of gastric ulcers[52]. Current recommendations are to test for and treat *H. pylori* infection in all patients with peptic ulcers[53]. Although there are several methods for diagnosing *H. pylori* infection, the urea breath tests are the most commonly used both to diagnose active infection and as a measure of success after eradication treatment[54].

Helicobacter pylori possesses the enzyme urease, which hydrolyses urea, releasing CO_2, which is then excreted in breath. Measuring CO_2 after giving the patient a labelled urea solution therefore allows a diagnosis of *H. pylori* infection to be made with a sensitivity of about 90-100 per cent and a specificity of about 78-100 per cent[55].

$$[NH_4]_2CO + H_2O \xrightarrow{\text{urease}} 2NH_3 + CO_2 + 2H_2$$

Urea is labelled with either ^{13}C or ^{14}C. The ^{14}C isotope has a small dose of radioactivity and requires special handling. The samples need to be sent to specialized laboratories for analysis; the use of this isotope is unsuitable in pregnant women and babies. The isotope ^{13}C is stable and the test is safe and easy to perform. Assay of ^{13}C is carried out usually by atomic absorption and many commercial laboratories offer this service.

Test protocol

The patient is asked to fast for at least 4-6 hours before the test. The patient should not have received antibiotics, bismuth or proton pump inhibitors for at least 2 weeks before the test.

Breath samples are taken at baseline, and 10-30 min after taking the test substance, which includes labelled urea. The samples are analysed for CO_2 and results are expressed qualitatively.

Interpretation

Test results are usually expressed as either positive or negative for *H. pylori* infection. False-negative tests can occur if the patient is on the drugs mentioned above. False-positive tests usually occur in the presence of achlorhydria or if the test is performed too soon (< 4 weeks) after eradication treatment is given.

Other, less common uses

Radiolabelled fatty acids and esters have been described in the assessment of pancreatic exocrine function[56, 57]. After absorption, the labelled fatty acid is metabolized to $^{14}CO_2$ in the liver and can be detected in the breath. These tests are affected by various factors and therefore have a very low sensitivity.

^{14}C-labelled glycocholic acid has been used to identify bile salt malabsorption in some patients with diarrhoea[58]. However, this test is technically difficult to perform and has a high false-positive rate.

The aminopyrine breath test, in which $^{14}CO_2$ is measured in breath after administering labelled methyl aminopyrine, has been described in the assessment of quantitative liver function[59].

Conclusion

Over the last three decades breath tests have been gradually introduced in the investigation and management of patients with various gastrointestinal disorders. Most breath tests are based on a simple physiological principle, involving metabolism of an ingested substrate by bacteria, thus releasing a gas that can be reliably detected in the breath. Currently, breath testing is most useful in the diagnosis of lactose malabsorption, bacterial overgrowth syndromes and *Helicobacter pylori* infection. It is non-invasive, relatively cheap and in most cases reliable. As the technology improves in the future, leading to improved specificity, it is likely that the indications for and use of breath testing will become more widespread.

References

1. Newcomer AD, McGill DB, Thomas PJ, Hofman AF. Prospective comparison indirect methods of detecting lactase deficiency. N Engl J Med 1975; 293: 1232-1236
2. Bond JH, Levitt MD. Quantitative measurement of lactose absorption. Gastroenterology 1976; 70: 1058-1062
3. Douwes AC, Fernandes J, Deenhart HJ. Improved accuracy of lactose tolerance test in children using expired H_2 measurement. Arch Dis Child 1978; 53: 939-942
4. Kneepkens CM, Vonk RJ, Fernandez J. Incomplete intestinal absorption of fructose. Arch Dis Child 1984; 59: 735-738
5. Gudmand-Hyer E, Krasilnikoff PA, Skovbjerg H. Sucrose-isomaltose malabsorption. Adv Nutr Res 1984; 6: 233-269
6. Davidson GP, Robb TA. Detection of primary and secondary sucrose malabsorption in children by means of the breath hydrogen technique. Med J Aust 1983; 2: 29-32
7. Metz G, Gassull MA, Drasr BS, Jenkins DJ, Blendis LM. Breath hydrogen test for small intestinal bacterial colonisation. Lancet 1976; i: 668-669
8. Rhodes JM, Middleton P, Jewell DP. The lactulose hydrogen breath test as a diagnostic tool for small bowel bacterial overgrowth. Scand J Gastroenterol 1979; 14: 333-336
9. Diggory RT, Cuschieri A. The effect of dose and osmolality of lactulose on the oral-caecal transit time determined by the hydrogen breath test and the reproducibility of the test in normal subjects. Ann Clin Res 1985; 17: 331-333
10. Bjrneklett A, Jenssen E. Relationship between hydrogen and methane production in man. Scand J Gastroenterol 1982; 17: 985-992
11. Fritz M, Siebert G, Kasper H. Dose dependence of breath hydrogen and methane in healthy volunteers after ingestion of a commercial disaccharide mixture, Palatinit. Br J Nutr 1985; 54: 389-400
12. Marshall BJ, Warren JR. Unidentified curved bacilli in the stomach of patients with gastritis and peptic ulceration. Lancet 1984; i: 311-315
13. Feldman ME, Fieldman LS, Sleisenger MH. Gastrointestinal and Liver Disease, 6th edn. New York: Saunders, 2002
14. Levitt MD, Hirsh P, Fetzer CA, Sheahan M, Levine AS. H_2 excretion after ingestion of complex carbohydrates. Gastroenterology 1987; 92: 383-389
15. Stephen AM. Starch and dietary fiber: their physiological and epidemiological interrelationships. Can J Physiol Pharmacol 1991; 69: 116-120
16. Strocchi A, Levitt MD. Measurement of starch absorption in humans. Can J Physiol Pharmacol 1991; 69: 108-110
17. Peerman JA, Modler S. Glycoproteins as substrates for production of hydrogen and methane by colonic bacterial flora. Gastroenterology 1982; 83: 388-393
18. Pitzalis G, Fancellu MG, Degnelloll F, Galstri E, Bonamico M, Imperatol C. Prevalence of lactose malabsorption in Roman schoolchildren. An H_2 breath study using cows' milk. Minerva Paediatr 1993; 45: 389-395

19. Brummer RJ, Armbrecht U, Bosaeus I, Dotevail G, Stockbruegger RW. The hydrogen breath test. Sampling methods and the influence of dietary fibre on fasting level. Scand J Gastroenterol 1985; 20: 1007-1013

20. Davidson GP, Robb TA. Value of breath hydrogen analysis management of diarrhoeal illness in childhood: comparison with duodenal biopsy. J Paediatr Gastroenterol Nutr 1985; 4: 381-387

21. Fernandes J, Vos CE, Douwes AC, Slotema E, Degenhart HJ. Respiratory hydrogen excretion as a parameter for lactose malabsorption in children. Am J Clin Nutr 1978; 31: 597-602

22. Filali A, Ben Hassine L, Dhouib H, Matri S, Ben Ammar A, Garoui H. Study of malabsorption of lactose by the H_2 breath test in a population of 70 Tunisian adults. Gastroenterol Clin Biol 1987; 11: 554-557

23. Douwes AC, Schaap C, Van Der Kleivan Moorsel JM. Hydrogen breath test in schoolchildren. Arch Dis Child 1985; 60: 333-337

24. Gilat T, Ben Hur H, Gelman-Malachi E, Terdiman R, Peled Y. Alterations of the colonic flora and their effect on the hydrogen breath test. Gut 1978; 19: 602-605

25. Solomons NW, Garcia R, Schneider R, Viteri FE, Von Kaenel VA. H_2 breath tests during diarrhoea. Acta Paediatr Scand 1979; 88: 171-172

26. Cloarec D, Bornet F, Gouilloud S, Barry JL, Galmiche JP. Breath hydrogen response to lactulose in healthy subjects: relationship to methane producing status. Gut 1990; 31: 300-304

27. Robb TA, Goodwin DA, Davidson GP. Faecal hydrogen production in vitro as an indicator for in vivo hydrogen producing capability in the hydrogen breath test. Acta Paediatr Scand 1985; 74: 942-944

28. Solomons NW. Evaluation of carbohydrate absorption: the hydrogen breath test in clinical practice. Clin Nutr J 1984; 3: 71-78

29. Goldin E, Wengrower D. Diarrhoea in hypothyroidism: bacterial overgrowth as a possible aetiology. J Clin Gastroenterol 1990; 12: 98-99

30. Davidson GP, Robb TA, Kirubakaran CP. Bacterial contamination of the small intestine as an important cause of chronic diarrhoea and abdominal pain: diagnosis by breath hydrogen test. Paediatrics 1984; 74: 229-235

31. Sherr HP, Sasaki Y, Newman A et al. Detection of bacterial deconjugation of bile salts by a convenient breath-analysis technique. N Engl J Med 1975; 285: 656

32. Casellas F, Chicharro L, Malagelada JR. Potential usefulness of hydrogen breath test with D-xylose in clinical management of intestinal malabsorption. Dig Dis Sci 1993; 38; 321-327

33. Corazza GR, Menozzi MG, Strocchi A et al. The diagnosis of small bowel bacterial overgrowth. Reliability of jejunal culture and inadequacy of breath hydrogen testing. Gastroenterology 1990; 98: 302-309

34. Riordan SM, McIver CJ, Walker BM, Duncombe VM, Bolin TD, Thomas MC. The lactulose breath test and small intestinal bacterial overgrowth. Am J Gastroenterol 1996; 91: 1795-1803

35. King CE, Toskes PP. Comparison of the 1-gram [^{14}C]xylose, 10-gram lactulose-H_2, and 80-gram glucose-H_2 breath tests in patients with small intestinal bacterial overgrowth. Gastroenterology 1986; 91: 1447-1451

36. Perman JA, Modler S, Barr RG, Rosenthal P. Fasting breath hydrogen concentration: normal values and clinical application. Gastroenterology 1984; 87: 1358-1363

37. Corazza GR, Strocchi A, Gasbarrini G. Fasting breath hydrogen in coeliac disease. Gastroenterology 1997; 93: 53-58

38. Kerlin P, Wong L. Breath hydrogen testing in bacterial overgrowth of the small intestine. Gastroenterology 1998; 95: 982-988

39. Labrooy SJ, Male PJ, Beavis AK, Misiewicz JJ. Assessment of the reproducibility of the lactulose H_2 breath test as a measure of mouth to caecum transit time. Gut 1983; 24: 893-896

40. Camboni G, Basilisco G, Bozzani A, Bianchi PA. Repeatability of lactulose hydrogen breath test in subjects with normal or prolonged oro-caecal transit. Dig Dis Sci 1988; 33: 1525-1527

41. Jorge JM, Wexner SD, Ehrenpreis ED. The lactulose hydrogen breath test as a measure of oro-caecal transit time. Eur J Surg 1994; 160: 409-416

42. Wilberg S, Pieramico O, Malfertheiner P. The H_2-lactulose breath test in the diagnosis of intestinal transit time. Leber Magen Darm 1990; 20: 129-137

43. Murphy MS, Nelson R, Eastham EJ. Measurement of small intestinal transit time in children. Acta Paediatr Scand 1988; 77: 802-806

44. Dalzell AM, Freestone NS, Billington D, Heaf DP. Small intestinal permeability and oro-caecal transit time in cystic fibrosis. Arch Dis Child 1990; 65: 585-588

45. Gotze H, Ptok A. Oro-caecal transit time in patients with Crohn's disease. Eur J Paediatr 1993; 152: 193-196

46. Basilisco G, Camboni G, Bozzan Y, Vita P, Doldi S, Bianchi PA. Oro-caecal transit delay in obese patients. Dig Dis Sci 1989; 34: 509-512

47. Scott AM, Kellow JE, Eckersley GM, Nolan JM, Jones MP. Cigarette smoking and nicotine delay postprandial mouth-caecum transit time. Dig Dis Sci 1993; 37: 1544-1547

48. Gorard DA, Gomborone JE, Libby GW, Farthing MJ. Intestinal transit in anxiety and depression. Gut 1996; 39: 551-555

49. Lawson M, Kern F Jr, Everson GT. Gastrointestinal transit time in human pregnancy: prolongation in the second and third trimesters followed by postpartum normalisation. Gastroenterology 1985; 89: 996-999

50. Szilagyi A, Salomon R, Martin M, Fokeeff K, Seidman E. Lactose handling by women with lactose malabsorption is improved during pregnancy. Clin Invest Med 1996; 19: 416-426

51. Bozzani A, Camboni MG, Tidone L et al. Gastrointestinal transit in hyperthyroid patients before and after propranolol treatment. Am J Gastroenterol 1985; 80: 550-552

52. National Institute of Health Consensus Conference. *Helicobacter pylori* in peptic ulcer disease. JAMA 1994; 272: 65-69

53. The European *Helicobacter pylori* Study Group. Current European concepts in the management of *Helicobacter pylori* infection. The Maastricht Consensus Report. Gut 1997; 48: 8-13

54. Atherton JC, Spiller RC. The urea breath test for *Helicobacter pylori*. Gut 1998; 43(suppl 1): 547-550

55. Goddard AF, Logan RPH. Review article: urea breath tests for detecting *Helicobacter pylori*. Aliment Pharmacol Ther 1997; 11: 641-649

56. Vantrappen GR, Rutgeerts PJ, Ghoos YF, Hiele MI. Mixed triglyceride breath test: a noninvasive test of pancreatic lipase activity in the duodenum. Gastroenterology 1989; 96: 1126

57. Cole SG, Rossi S, Stern A, Hoffmann AF. Cholesteryl octanoate breath test. Gastroenterology 1987; 93: 1372

58. Fromm H, Malavolti M. Bile acid induced diarrhoea. Clin Gastroenterol 1986; 15: 567-582

59. Jalan R, Hayes PC. Review article: Quantitative tests of liver function. Aliment Pharmacol Ther 1995; 9: 263

Chapter 5
Pathophysiological correlations in anorectal conditions

MICHAEL ER WILLIAMSON

The normal functioning of the anorectum is a complex interplay of anal and rectal sensation, muscle action, rectal capacitance and stool consistency[1]. An abnormality in any one, but certainly in any combination of these factors, may result in a disorder of defecation. Each component of the defecatory mechanism can be measured individually and specific defects identified; however, more important and difficult to measure is the coordinated action of the different components.

There are pressure receptors in the pelvic floor that detect rectal distension and these can be stimulated via distension of the rectum by balloons filled with air or water. Within the anal canal, especially the upper centimetre marking the transitional zone between anus and rectum, there is a high density of sensory endings that are capable of detecting touch and temperature. A combination of the sensory endings allows the differentiation of solid, liquid and gas, which is essential to appropriate social behaviour and determination of when to visit the toilet. Even in normal individuals this very clever mechanism can be fooled with sometimes embarrassing results. In stark contrast to their subtlety, the measurement of anal canal sensation is crude and usually by detection of an electrical pulse. It is, however, repeatable and therefore a reliable test.

The motor component of anorectal function consists of the involuntary internal anal sphincter and the voluntary external anal sphincter. The strength of these guardians of the anus can be measured by detecting the pressure that they produce within the anal canal, using probes attached to pressure monitors. At rest, the greatest component of contraction and therefore anal canal pressure is from the internal anal sphincter, and any reduction in

73

pressure at rest is usually the result of damage to that muscle. The external sphincter can be voluntarily recruited and is also the most active sphincter in reflex reaction to coughing and sneezing. Therefore, if anal canal pressure is measured when asking the patient to squeeze or cough, the extra pressure generated will usually reflect the external anal sphincter's ability to contract. Of course there must also be pressure generated within the colon and rectum to promote normal evacuation and these synchronized peristaltic waves can be measured using pressure sensors mounted on wires placed within the rectum and colon. These tests of colonic motility are not widely available and are useful only as research tools.

The capacitance of the rectum is an essential component in allowing a normal bowel action. The effect on continence of a low capacitance rectum can be observed in patients with inflammatory bowel disease. These patients, who have normal sensation and normal or heightened muscle strength, must cope with urgency and sometimes incontinence because their rectum has been scarred by repeated inflammation and can no longer stretch. Distending an intrarectal balloon with air or water can mimic rectal filling. The pressure required to distend the rectum reveals its compliance, whereas the sensation may be reported by the patient or witnessed as causing reflex inhibition of the anal sphincter - the rectoanal inhibitory reflex.

Faecal incontinence

Relevant investigations[2] of this are:

- Anal manometry
- Rectoanal inhibitory reflex
- Anal canal sensation
- Pudendal nerve terminal motor latency
- Electromyography (EMG)
- Endoanal ultrasonography.

Incontinence of faeces is a surprisingly common problem that usually results from weakness in the internal anal sphincter, the external anal sphincter or a combination of both. Some people with entirely normal anal sphincters may occasionally be incontinent of faeces when the normal systems are stretched beyond their considerable reserve, e.g. when stressed by the watery diarrhoea associated with infective or idiopathic inflammatory bowel disease. Some patients will report incontinence when in fact they have the less troublesome condition of faecal soiling. This distinction needs to be made because patients who report faecal soiling of their underwear, often associated with pruritis ani, may on testing have longer than normal anal sphincters and higher than average pressures when manometry is performed. A common association is haemorrhoids, and all patients require is simple treatment for the haemorrhoids, a healthier diet and advice about managing their pruritis.

The importance of a thorough history that includes diet, medications, previous endoanal surgery, perineal surgery or childbirth cannot be stressed enough. In particular, an obstetric history recording a difficult, prolonged labour and/or vaginal delivery resulting in a significant perineal tear, especially if forceps were required, may identify the origins of incontinence. The time of onset of incontinence recalled by the patient may not necessarily be at the time of probable damage.

For many years the standard investigation for faecal incontinence was the measurement of anal canal pressure at rest and during voluntary contraction (squeeze) or cough, and the measurement of anal canal sensation. It is important that any measurement of pressure or sensation is compared with the normal values for the same laboratory because the results may vary significantly between laboratories. A reduced resting anal pressure implies a defect of the internal anal sphincter, whereas a reduced squeeze or cough increment implies a defect in the external sphincter (usually accompanied by a lower than normal resting pressure). Poor anal canal pressures, both at rest and during squeeze, imply a deficiency in both sphincters and are likely to be associated with severe incontinence.

Although the existence of a sphincter abnormality can be identified by anal manometry, and even correlated with a history of damage, it is not possible to identify the underlying pathological process causing the weakness using these techniques. For example, in a patient with a history of prolonged labour ending in a forceps delivery and third-degree perineal tear, sphincter weakness could be caused by an anatomical defect from direct trauma or neurological damage from pudendal nerve stretching and secondary muscle weakness. The differentiation is important because anatomical defects can be repaired surgically whereas damaged nerves cannot. Surgery is likely to be a failure and therefore at best a waste of time and money. Early attempts to image sphincter muscle structure involved using multiple pressure transducers arranged around the circumference of the anal canal (vector volumes) or mapping the electrical signals of the muscles (EMG). Using either technique, a crude impression of muscle integrity could be achieved; however, it was the advent of an ultrasound machine that could scan the anal muscles accurately that provided the real answer.

Unarguably, the most important recent advance in the investigation of faecal incontinence is endoanal ultrasonography (see Chapter 9). A rotating ultrasound transducer is mounted on a rod that can be inserted into the anal canal or rectum. The various layers of the anal canal, including the internal and external anal sphincters, can be seen clearly as dark (hypoechoic) and light (hyperechoic) rings, respectively. Perineal trauma resulting in even minimal division of a sphincter will allow the muscle ends to pull widely apart. The intervening scar tissue that develops appears different to the normal muscle and therefore a defect in the internal anal sphincter, the external anal sphincter or both sphincters can usually be visualized on endoanal ultrasonography. Although it is useful to document any alteration of anal canal pressure, it is the appearance of the sphincters on imaging that is most likely to determine the cause of the incontinence or measured weakness and the likelihood of successful repair. One would expect some correlation with the patient history to explain the origin of a sphincter tear – either a significant perineal tear (third degree implies involving the anal sphincters) or previous anal trauma including planned surgical procedures. If identified, good results can be achieved by surgical repair of the anal sphincter.

The definition of the endoanal ultrasound image allows for the measurement of internal and external sphincter thickness, and average values have been recorded for normal individuals. One should be aware that there is a wide variation in the ultrasound anatomy of the anal canal between normal individuals. When scanning a weak anal sphincter complex, rather than an obvious muscle defect, a narrow, atrophic-looking sphincter may be revealed. If the internal anal sphincter is thin, it usually implies a primary degeneration, often associated with increasing age. A thin and atrophic external anal sphincter is most likely to result from denervation because of damage to the pudendal nerves.

If pudendal nerve damage is suspected, the nerve itself (one on each side) can be assessed by electrophysiological tests. Although the motor component of the pudendal nerve controls the external sphincter, the sensory component is responsible for sensation within the anal canal. The sensitivity of the anal canal can be measured by the detection of a small pulsating current applied to the mucosa and skin. A decreased anal canal sensation may help to confirm that the pudendal nerves are damaged, but it is a crude measure. More specialist electrophysiological tests are required to confirm pudendal nerve damage. Perhaps the best method is to measure the pudendal nerve terminal motor latency. A finger-mounted electrode both stimulates and records the response of the pudendal nerve, and any delay in the response compared with normal reveals nerve damage. A less direct, more difficult and more painful technique is to stick minute electrodes into the external anal sphincter (EMG) and to measure the tiny electrical signals arriving from the pudendal nerve. A damaged nerve produces a characteristic pattern. If either of these tests identifies pudendal nerve damage, then a careful history may elicit the aetiology. Persistent straining at stool for many years will result in stretching and damage of the nerve. Damage may also result from relatively short but intense periods of stretching and direct pressure experienced during a protracted and difficult labour. It is important to identify pudendal nerve damage, but unfortunately there is no surgical solution to the problem. The concurrence of pudendal nerve damage and sphincter muscle tears is important to identify, because it is likely that surgical repair of the sphincter defect will have a poorer result than in the presence of normal nerve function. There now seems to be hope for reasonable recovery of function associated with the new procedure of sacral nerve neuromodulation.

For some patients, a complaint of incontinence may actually underlie a diagnosis of constipation. Particularly in the elderly patient, a lack of rectal sensation may lead to rectal distension with faeces. The result is 'overflow' of the faecal bolus by liquid motion, which leaks through a weak anal sphincter. Although it is likely that a global problem in association with decreased rectal sensation causes the decreased sphincter tone, it has also been postulated that the internal anal sphincter relaxes because of reflex inhibition from the presence of a large faecal bolus. No fancy investigations are required – a simple digital examination will reveal the cause and allow correction before considering investigation of the constipation (see below). Interestingly, this relationship between rectal distension by faeces and reflex sphincter relaxation causing soiling/incontinence is also observed in children with chronic constipation, although it usually improves if the constipation continues into adulthood, to be replaced by discomfort.

Rectal prolapse with incontinence

Relevant investigations for this are:

- Anal manometry
- Rectoanal inhibitory reflex
- Anal canal sensation
- Pudendal nerve terminal motor latency
- Endoanal ultrasonography
- Defecating proctogram.

Rectal prolapse can be subdivided into partial- and full-thickness prolapse. Partial-thickness prolapse occurs when redundant folds of excess mucosal lining descend from the lower rectum and through the anus on straining. Usually, mucosal prolapse occurs in the anterior midline (anterior mucosal prolapse), but it can involve increasing amounts up to the full circumference. Such a prolapse rarely involves more than a few centimetres of prolapse beyond the anal verge, and to the trained examining fingers it is thin, consisting of only a double layer of mucosa and submucosa. Partial prolapse probably results from repeated straining and can be difficult to dissociate from prolapsing haemorrhoids. Although patients with partial prolapse may describe 'incontinence', it usually amounts to no more than soiling and mucus discharge. Anal manometry will usually reveal normal or only slightly low resting (internal anal) sphincter pressures. Anal canal sensation, on the other hand, is usually reduced but this reflects the downward displacement of the sensitive zone more than any nerve dysfunction. Endoanal ultrasonography may reveal thickened lower rectal mucosa caused by the oedema and fibrous reaction in the prolapsing mucosa. Resolution of the prolapse using rubber band ligation or injection of sclerosant is effective in eradicating the symptoms. It is also possible that the new procedure of stapled mucosectomy may offer good quality symptom resolution.

Full-thickness rectal prolapse is a far more debilitating condition, resulting from the complete prolapse of the full-thickness rectum. Although the patient may describe a thick prolapse extending for 4–10 cm beyond the anal verge, there may be relatively little to see on examination; on straining, however, marked pelvic floor descent with bright red mucosa appearing at the anus is typical. The prolapse usually occurs after defecation and initially returns by itself. With time the patient needs to replace the prolapse and eventually it will not return at all without medical help. If clinically suspected, but difficult to demonstrate, a full-thickness rectal prolapse can best be diagnosed by a defecating proctogram. In this radiological test, paste containing radiologically active contrast is introduced into the rectum and the patient is asked to pass the paste while sitting on a commode before the X-ray machine. The prolapse is usually clearly seen starting as an intussusception high in the rectum, prolapsing through the anus in gross cases. This method is particularly sensitive at detecting rectal prolapse that does not clinically protrude beyond the anus.

Although chronic constipation and straining are the most common cause of full-thickness rectal prolapse, many patients report incontinence to faeces. There are a number of possible reasons for incontinence and these vary between individuals. The real problem lies in whether or not the repeated straining that led to the prolapse has also caused pudendal nerve damage. If nerve damage has occurred, the anal sphincter complex will be irretrievably weakened and incontinence is likely to persist after repair of the rectal prolapse. If the pudendal nerves are intact, the anal sphincter complex may show reduced pressures on manometry because of the persistence of prolapsing tissue in the anal canal. Furthermore, the presence of prolapsing upper rectum lying within the lower rectum, in addition to causing tenesmus (a persistent feeling of need to pass stool detected by the patient), causes reflex inhibition of the internal anal sphincter (the rectoanal inhibitory reflex) and reduced anal canal pressure. Both of these effects, mainly on the internal anal sphincter, can be reversed by appropriate surgical repair of the prolapse. Patients with rectal prolapse who have reduced anal squeeze pressures (external anal sphincter) and evidence of prolonged pudendal nerve terminal motor latency are likely to remain incontinent after operation. Patients with reduced resting anal pressures (internal anal sphincter) and normal pudendal nerve terminal motor latency may expect improved incontinence after operation, but this is by no means guaranteed. In practice, because of the lack of availability of motor latency measurements for the pudendal nerve and the relatively imprecise nature of sphincter pressure measurements, it is wise to avoid operations that result in looser bowel motions in the presence of clinical incontinence or measurable reduction in anal canal pressures.

Constipation

Relevant investigations for this are:

- Barium enema
- Colonic transit study (gastric emptying study)

- Rectal sensation (anal manometry)
- Rectoanal inhibitory reflex
- Defecating proctogram
- Balloon expulsion
- EMG.

It is important to define constipation because the term means different things to different patients and different doctors[3]. Constipation may be used to describe difficulty in passing large hard stools or, alternatively, it may be used to describe infrequent defecation, often associated with bloating and pain. Decreased frequency and hard stools usually coexist and can be correlated to an increased time for faeces to pass through the colon and rectum (colonic transit time), leading to an increase in fluid resorption and a decrease in bacterial content. Dietary fibre with adequate fluid intake increases stool bulk and bacterial content, and reduces colonic transit time. Many normal individuals report constipation on occasions but, for the purposes of the following section, I refer only to persistent chronic constipation as a recognized disease. A normal frequency of bowel action is said to be between three stools a day and one stool every 3 days; however, most people agree that a good starting point for a definition of chronic constipation is someone who passes hard stool less than once a week. 'Constipation' of any degree less than this rather strict definition will usually respond to simple measures, especially increasing fibre and fluid intake for a decent period of time, or by introducing laxatives. These simple measures certainly should precede any investigation of a person presenting with constipation for the first time.

When investigating and treating constipation, it is important to rule out any anatomical abnormality of the colon or rectum such as a stricture caused by malignant or benign disease. Although such a cause is unlikely in someone presenting with a long history of constipation, in addition to excluding disease a barium enema examination may reveal more subtle abnormalities including distended bowel (megacolon or megarectum) or an abnormally long colon (less easy to define). If an anatomical abnormality or external influence (dietary, endocrine or other medical disease) has been excluded, two main types of constipation are recognized. In slow transit constipation the normal colonic peristaltic waves responsible for moving faeces to the rectum are defective. This may be true for the whole colon, in which case it is sometimes associated with a panenteric (whole gastrointestinal tract from pharynx to rectum) neuromuscular disorder, or one part of the colon. If, on the other hand, colonic motility is normal but the patient cannot empty the rectum the term 'obstructive defecation' has been applied. Although there is no true anatomical obstruction, some patients seem to display a functional outlet (anus) obstruction to the passage of even liquid faeces, and hence the obstructive label has been widely applied. It is of paramount importance to differentiate between the two conditions because the treatment is different for each; unfortunately, however, the two may coexist in the same patient, making management particularly difficult.

Megacolon and megarectum are diagnosed by the appearance of distended colon on a barium enema examination (specifically the width of the rectosigmoid at the pelvic brim). A well-known, but in truth rare, cause for this is Hirschsprung's disease, in which there is an embryological failure of development of nerve cells in the rectal wall. This causes a permanently contracted segment of rectum and colon with distended colon above it. Rarely, patients with a particularly short segment of Hirschsprung's disease can reach adulthood with apparently simple chronic constipation, but if the disease is suspected it can be revealed by one of two tests. The nerves that fail to develop in Hirschsprung's disease are the nerves that subserve the rectoanal inhibitory reflex and, therefore, if the reflex is absent in association with constipation there is a high chance that Hirschsprung's disease is the cause. A more definitive but invasive test is to perform full-thickness rectal biopsy and look for the presence or absence of nerve cells under the microscope.

The only treatment for Hirschsprung's disease is surgical bypass of the non-working segment of the colon and rectum. In cases of very short segment disease, one can often get away with standard treatments for chronic constipation.

Slow transit constipation

Implicit in the name, this type of constipation appears to result from the inability of the colon to transfer the faeces along the colon to the rectum, from where it may be expelled. Highly specialized experiments, in which pressure transducers are placed along the length of the colon, reveal different patterns of contractile activity in normal and constipated individuals. In normal individuals there are frequent low-amplitude non-propagating contractions, but occasionally there are also high-amplitude contractions that propagate along the colon to the rectum, some of which stimulate defecation. They usually occur in the morning after waking and sometimes after meals, and can be initiated by stimulant laxatives.

In many patients with idiopathic constipation, such propagated activity is less frequent and of lower amplitude, and rarely results in defecation. In many of these patients, stimulant laxatives also fail to initiate the high-pressure contractions. In addition to these physiological studies, microscopic examination has revealed subtle abnormalities of the nerve fibres in the colonic wall of constipated patients. However, similar changes can be seen in experimental animals after prolonged administration of stimulant laxatives, and the changes may therefore be induced by treatment, rather than be the cause of the constipation.

Leaving aside specialized tests, the standard investigation for suspected slow transit constipation is to perform a colonic transit study. In its most simple form, the patient is asked to swallow some radiological marker beads and their progress along the colon is observed by repeat radiograph. Initially the protocol included a radiograph soon after marker ingestion, to check that the markers had indeed been swallowed, but hopefully this is not required in most cases. The number of follow-up radiographs is usually reduced to a single film on day 5. In normal individuals nearly all the markers should be absent from the abdomen by this time. If most of the markers have not even reached the rectum, slow transit constipation is diagnosed and the segment of colon beyond the apparent hold-up of the markers should be the dysfunctional bowel. If all the markers have reached the rectum, but have not been evacuated, it would support, although not prove, a diagnosis of obstructed defecation. One drawback with the colonic transit study is that a false result can be obtained if the markers are held up artificially in the proximal colon by the effects of gross faecal loading from a distal obstruction. In this circumstance, slow transit constipation might be diagnosed when in fact the cause is obstructed defecation. Therefore, an attempt to exclude obstructive defecation should always accompany the transit study (see below).

If the markers are held up in the right colon, it is useful to perform at least a gastric emptying study to exclude a panenteric motility problem. In some patients the markers may be held up in the left colon or 'hindgut'. Left-sided constipation typically may be described by a patient who reports onset of constipation after a pelvic operation, childbirth, or lower spinal and sacral trauma. Experiments have revealed a failure of propagated waves and microscopic abnormalities of colonic nerve fibres in these patients. It is believed that autonomic nerve damage is responsible and that excision of the left colon will have a favourable result in this situation.

Some centres offer a radioisotope colonic transit study. Although more costly and more time-consuming, it is claimed that this type of transit study is more accurate at identifying segmental delay, perhaps allowing for treatment of a segment rather than the whole colon.

When medical treatments have failed, a surgical solution to slow transit constipation is to excise the whole colon and join the small bowel to the rectum. This procedure is not without side effects, is ineffective for relief of pain associated with constipation and, in the presence of a panenteric disorder, will almost certainly fail with time.

Obstructive defecation

This terminology arose because investigators discovered that, in some patients, constipation occurred because the voluntary muscles of the anus, instead of relaxing, were abnormally contracting during attempts to defecate and therefore causing a functional obstruction. This 'paradoxical' contraction was also called anismus. The puborectalis muscle is the uppermost of the external anal sphincter and forms a sling at the anorectal junction. Paradoxical contraction of this particular voluntary muscle results in a failure of the anorectal junction to straighten, making the passage of even soft faeces very difficult. EMG studies use fine electrodes passed through the skin of the perineum and into the muscle fibres of puborectalis. When normal individuals are asked to defecate, the electrical signals within the muscle subside as the muscle relaxes, but in patients with obstructed defecation the electrical signals actually increase as the muscle contracts. If EMG of the external anal sphincter is performed, a similar phenomenon is observed. EMG is a highly specialized investigation, not available in most anorectal laboratories, but the contracting muscle can easily be palpated and even seen during a defecating proctogram as an indentation at the top of the anal canal posteriorly. Unfortunately, after the initial interest in this phenomenon, it was noted that some normal individuals displayed the same paradoxical contractions under laboratory conditions whereas some patients diagnosed with obstructive defecation no longer displayed paradoxical contraction if ambulatory pressure studies were performed in the home environment. Therefore the true cause of 'obstructive defecation' is less clear, although there is no doubt that the phenomenon of paradoxical contraction is more prevalent among patients who complain of constipation. It may simply be a learned response to repeated straining to empty the rectum. When examining these patients, the abnormal muscle contraction is often associated with excessive descent of the pelvic floor, and the most likely explanation for obstructive defecation is a loss of the normal complex coordination between muscle groups.

These problems can most usefully be investigated by asking patients to pass standard objects. It is of interest that individuals reporting an entirely normal ability to defecate find considerable difficulty in trying to pass even small objects, if they are hard. This underlines the importance of achieving a soft stool before contemplating investigation. Normal individuals should experience little difficulty in expelling a 50-ml balloon filled with water. Patients with obstructed defecation, on the other hand, may find difficulty in expelling liquid itself, let alone liquid within a balloon. This balloon expulsion test can be useful in identifying a group of patients with obstructive defecation, and their later ability to expel balloons of increasing volume can be used to test their response to treatment.

Anorectal manometry is of limited use in diagnosing obstructive defecation, but knowledge of normal anal canal pressures is useful, and the presence of an anorectal inhibitory reflex excludes the possibility of Hirschsprung's disease. Manometry may be useful in identifying a group of patients whose failure to defecate appears to be caused by a lack of rectal sensation. Distension of a balloon filled with water or air will cause an increasing desire to defecate in normal individuals. The balloon may first be detected at quite small volumes of around 20–40 ml; later the experiment has to be stopped because of an intense and painful desire to defecate called the maximum tolerated volume. Some patients with constipation reveal, on testing, that they have a poor ability to sense rectal distension but a relatively normal maximum tolerated volume. It is believed that, by the time they perceive the need to defecate, the faecal bolus is too large. This condition is typical of old age.

There is no surgical solution for obstructive defecation. Early attempts to relax the paradoxical contraction of puborectalis and the external sphincter by surgical division failed, underlining the lack of direct cause of paradoxical contraction in the aetiology of the condition. Worse still, the division of the muscles resulted in incontinence combined with constipation. More modern techniques of chemical inhibition of paradoxical contraction have also failed to correct the disorder. Instead, the techniques that have been found to be of most benefit in obstructive defecation centre on restoring the coordination of the muscles of the anus and pelvic floor. The generic term for these interventions is 'biofeedback' and, in essence, they enable the patient to identify which muscles are responsible for defecation and, through retraining, allow them to relax. An effective method is to use anorectal manometry equipment attached to a large visual scale to allow the patients to observe when they are contracting puborectalis and the external anal sphincter, and then try to stop it. The results of biofeedback are variable, and very dependent on the time devoted to it and the attitudes of both the patient and the trainer to the technique.

Slow transit constipation with obstructed defecation

In patients who have evidence of obstructive defecation and an abnormal colonic transit study, it is important to remember that the transit study result may be false because of the effect of faecal hold-up. The treatment of choice for these patients is to perform biofeedback to cure the obstructive component and see if the patient is improved or cured. If biofeedback fails, it is important to repeat the colonic transit study to identify, after correction of the obstructive element, whether the patient displays idiopathic slow transit colon also. This component can then be managed as for any idiopathic slow transit constipation, as discussed above.

Failure to identify the obstructive component and perform surgical correction of slow transit constipation will almost certainly result in failure.

Rectocele

When performing defecating proctograms to investigate chronic constipation, it is not unusual to observe an anterior rectocele. They are far more common in women than in men and appear as a herniation of the mid and lower rectum forwards into the vagina. Some patients may describe this phenomenon clinically, being aware of a bulge into the lower vagina and even through the introitus during straining. When observing the proctogram one can see that the effort of straining diverts the faeces forward into the vagina instead of out through the anus. Some patients learn to correct this by applying digital pressure to the vaginal lump, which allows them successfully to pass stool. It is most likely that a rectocele is the result of long-term constipation rather than the cause, but its eradication can be helpful in restoring a patient's ability to defecate and then, by improving the constipation, prevent recurrence. Those competent in endoanal ultrasonography claim to be able to image the thin, atrophic anovaginal septum associated with the herniating rectum, but the definitive test remains the defecating proctogram.

Miscellaneous pathologies causing an elevation of anal canal pressure

Haemorrhoids are associated with higher than normal pressures, although there is much overlap. Typical symptoms include spots of fresh blood on the toilet paper after defecation and symptoms of pruritis ani (itchy anus). Haemorrhoidectomy by any method is usually associated with a decrease in resting pressure to normal.

Fissure *in ano* is a painful condition in which a split develops in the skin of the anal canal, usually the posterior midline. Reflex spasm of the anal sphincter further reduces an already poor blood supply to that region, preventing healing. Spots of fresh blood are also typically described but it is the severe pain, classically during defecation and for 30 minutes after, that differentiates it from haemorrhoids. The pain usually prevents per anal examination but, when this can be achieved, especially in more chronic cases, elevation of resting sphincter pressure is often reported. The cure for fissure *in ano* is to weaken the internal anal sphincter artificially, preferably by drugs, but in resistant cases the muscle may need to be surgically partially divided.

Conclusion

Using a combination of a careful patient history and appropriate investigations it is usually possible to identify the underlying cause for a disorder of defecation. Repeating the investigations after intervention may reveal a satisfactory improvement, consistent with improved clinical function, or the disorder may remain unchanged, confirming the reason for failure. Such correlation may also be absent, the patient reporting clinical improvement but no significant alteration of measurements. Some of the investigative techniques themselves may be of use for treatments, such as biofeedback.

The correction of defecatory disorders often presents a challenge, and as much information as possible is desirable to avoid unnecessary surgery and best inform the patient about the likelihood of improvement.

References

1. Pemberton JH, Swash M, Henry MM. The Pelvic Floor. London: Saunders-Harcourt, 2002
2. Smith LE. Practical Guide to Anorectal Testing. Tokyo: Igaku Shoin, 1995
3. Kamm M, Lennard-Jones JE. Constipation. Wrightson, 1994

Chapter 6
Anorectal physiology

RIDZUAN FAROUK

Standardized tests of physiological measurement have been increasingly used for the objective appraisal of anorectal function. These methods allow for a better understanding of anorectal dysfunction. In addition, physiological measurements provide a means of explaining outcomes after treatment. Manometry, electrophysiology and radiological assessment represent the standard techniques used in the assessment of anorectal function.

Manometric assessment

This may be performed in a number of ways. Each method is subject to its own disadvantages. Methods available include water-filled perfusion catheters, water- or air-filled balloons, sleeve catheters and solid-state pressure transducers. (see Figure 6.1)

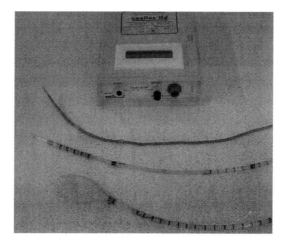

Figure 6.1 Types of manometry catheter: Ambulatory recorder; solid state; water perfused and rectal ballon catheters.

Perfused catheters

These catheters are usually multiport systems. Each port is perfused with water at a constant rate that is sufficient to keep the port open, but low enough to prevent errors arising because of anorectal filling. The pressure recorded in each port is an index of the resistance to flow of fluid out of the catheter. It has been reported that fluid leakage may result in sphincter contractions. Large-bore catheters may also record falsely high pressures. In addition, perfusion systems are dependent on the compliance of the system and the rate of perfusion. These systems are simple and relatively cheap to use. Computerized multiport analysis allows for three-dimensional imaging of the anal canal. In general, a lack of uniformity in materials and methods used has reduced the value of inter-unit comparisons of results.

Microballoon catheters

Similar alterations in anorectal contractility, as seen with perfused systems, may arise when using balloon systems. Large balloons are to be avoided because of the false increase in pressure. Balloon catheters avoid the potential artefacts caused by leakage, which is seen in perfused catheters, and are multidirectional rather than unidirectional. Air or water may be used with microballoon systems. Miller et al.[1] have shown good correlation between air- and water-filled systems, whereas Sun et al.[2] have shown the systems to be identical.

Sleeve catheters

Fluid is perfused through a sleeve formed by Silastic material glued over a Silastic base. In the anal canal, the sleeve spans the sphincter so that a contraction anywhere along its length will cause an increased resistance to the flow of fluid. This is measured as an increase in catheter pressure. The sleeve catheters are unable to distinguish between internal and external anal sphincter activity.

Microtransducers[3]

Microtransducers avoid many of the problems of perfused catheters by minimizing distension of the anus. They do, however, suffer from being unidirectional, fragile and expensive. They may be converted to an omnidirectional system by sealing the microtransducer in an air-filled microballoon. This increases the diameter of the probe, however, causing distension of the anus.

These transducers tend to be used for prolonged or ambulatory measurements.

Applications of manometry[4]

Manometry may be used for assessment of internal anal sphincter function (resting anal pressure), external sphincter function (maximum anal squeeze pressure), measurement of anal sphincter length[5] and the high-pressure zone of the anal canal, and for simple assessment of rectoanal integration (the rectoanal inhibitory reflex – discussed later).

Resting anal pressure

Tonic contraction of the internal anal sphincter (which consists of smooth muscle) is considered to contribute up to 85 per cent of the resting anal pressure. Normal resting anal pressure is dependent on whether the individual is alert or asleep, and on his or her position. Resting anal pressure in the 'normal' individual in the left lateral position is between 65 and 95 cmH$_2$O and increases by 25 per cent when the individual is ambulant. These values depend on age, parity and the absence of previous anal surgery. Basal resting pressure is not constant[6]. There are phasic variations called slow waves, which occur at a frequency of between 6/min and 20/min with an amplitude of 10–25 cmH$_2$O. Slow-wave frequency is higher in the distal anal canal and it is postulated that this provides a pressure gradient against possible incontinence during the sampling reflex (see later). In addition, ultra-slow waves with a frequency of 1–3/min and an amplitude of up to 100 cmH$_2$O also occur. Ultra-slow waves are more commonly observed in patients with chronic anal fissure and in those who suffer from chronic constipation.

Maximum anal sphincter squeeze pressure

Voluntary contraction of the external anal sphincter can be measured and is defined as the highest pressure recorded during maximum sphincter contraction. This is usually 50–100 per cent greater than resting anal pressure in normal individuals. The external anal sphincter consists of striated muscle (type 1 fibres) and is fatigable. Maximum voluntary squeeze pressure recordings may be supplemented in patients who have difficulty reproducing this manoeuvre in the left lateral position by measurement of the pressure obtained at coughing.

Pull-through measurement of anal canal length[7]

For the assessment of anal canal profile, the recording catheter must be withdrawn stepwise or continuously at a constant rate. The step-by-step pull-through technique at 30- to 60-second intervals provides reliable measurements of resting anal pressure. Anal sphincter length using this technique, based on the length of the zone of high pressure, is 2.5 ± 1 cm in men and 2.0 ± 1 cm in women. A slow, continuous pull-through represents a more appropriate method of assessing anal canal pressure profile and functional sphincter length. With this technique, anal sphincter length is considered to be 2.5-5 cm. The technique has been criticized, however, because it is considered to include a variable amount of reflex external anal sphincter contraction.

Anatomical, gender and age variability[8]

Intra-anal pressure exhibits longitudinal and radial variations. In the proximal part of the anal canal the pressure recorded in the dorsal segment is higher than the pressure in the anterior segment. This finding has been attributed to puborectalis muscle activity. In women, anal pressure in the anterior segment is higher distally, whereas in men the pressure is higher in the anterior and lateral segments proximally. The typical resting pressure profile during continuous pull-out describes the length and distribution of pressure along the longitudinal axis of the sphincter. The normal mean resting anal pressure ranges between 65 and 95 cmH$_2$O and is located 1.5-2 cm from the anal verge. The range of normal sphincter length based on pull-through techniques is 2.5-5 cm. Anal canal length tends to be greater in men because of the shorter length of the anterior axis of the anal canal in women.

Maximal squeeze pressures and sphincter length are greater in men compared with women. Mean resting anal pressure is comparable between men and nulliparous women. Parous women have lower mean resting anal pressure, lower maximal squeeze pressures and shorter sphincter length compared with nulliparous women. In addition, resting pressure, squeeze pressure and sphincter length all decrease with age.

Rectal function

Manometry may assist in the assessment of rectal reservoir function by infusing air or water at 37°C at a steady rate (60 ml/min) into a rectal balloon and comparing it with the rate of change of rectal pressure (rectal compliance)[9]. Initially the proctometrogram shows little or no increase in rectal pressure per unit of volume infused, but the rise in pressure becomes progressively steeper as the maximum tolerated volume is approached[10]. Volumes that it is valuable to record are the volume at first awareness, first sensation of the need to pass wind/defecate, the volume that induces urgency and the maximum tolerated volume. Initial perception of distension is usually noted during an initial rise in rectal pressure. There follows a plateau phase in the proctometrogram when most individuals will describe a sensation of wanting to pass flatus. The desire to defecate occurs at the onset of the final rapid ascent of rectal pressure. The tracing obtained provides for the estimation of rectal compliance, which is calculated by plotting volume versus pressure and calculating the gradient. Normal rectal compliance varies widely, between 4 and 14 ml/cmH$_2$O (see Figure 6.2). Suggested normal values are:

- First awareness: 40–70 ml
- First desire to defecate: 100–150 ml
- Urgency: 150–300 ml
- Maximum tolerated volume: 180–410 ml.

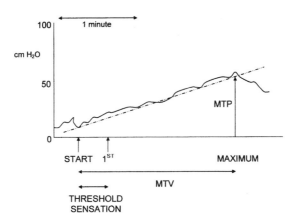

Figure 6.2 Rectal compliance from ano-rectal manometry.

Variability of rectal compliance, because of age, sex and/or the presence of faeces in the rectum, has previously been demonstrated[11]. A newer method using transrectal ultrasonography to measure rectal compliance has been described and mathematically validated[12]. Further studies will be required to assess its applicability.

A more accurate method of measuring rectal tone involves the insertion of a large-capacitance plastic bag into the rectum, filling the bag with water and connecting it to an external fluid reservoir. Rectal pressures are kept constant in this system while rectal volume is varied.

Patients with a space-occupying lesion of the rectum, e.g. rectal cancer or rectal prolapse, and those with an inflammatory process (inflammatory bowel disease or radiation injury), could be expected to have poor compliance and decreased thresholds to retaining saline. Patients with functional constipation appear to have poor rectal threshold to sensation and have increased rectal compliance. Patients with intractable constipation after hysterectomy also demonstrate poor rectal sensation in combination with increased rectal compliance.

The rectoanal inhibitory reflex

As the rectum is filled, the internal anal sphincter relaxes[13]. The laboratory demonstration of this phenomenon is likened to the physiological process of anal sampling, where the sensitive mucosa of the upper anal canal 'samples' rectal contents[14]. It can be detected using any of the previously mentioned manometry systems. It is most easily elicited by inflating a balloon attached to a Nelaton catheter via a three-way valve to a 50-ml Luer lock syringe. In normal individuals, the reflex is observed after instillation of 10–30 ml air and is followed by a desire to pass flatus after 40–50 ml instilled air. The reflex is absent in Hirschsprung's disease and can be used diagnostically for this purpose. Patients with rectal prolapse may not demonstrate the reflex – this is because the internal anal sphincter is submaximally inhibited via distension of the rectum by the presence of the prolapse within it. Patients who have undergone low anterior resection, coloanal anastomosis or ileoanal pouch surgery may not possess the reflex because of transsection of the descending inhibitory neurons in the distal rectum, which mediate the rectoanal inhibitory reflex.

Electromyography

Electromyography (EMG) has traditionally been one of the main investigative techniques used in the investigation of the anal sphincter and pelvic floor muscles[15]. Individual muscle fibres

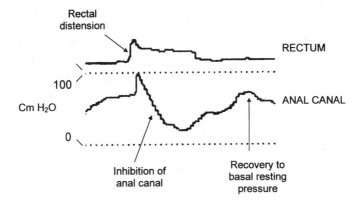

Figure 6.3 Rectoanal inhibition.

derived from a motor unit summate to form the motor unit action potential. This can be recorded at a greater distance than the close proximity that is required to record individual muscle fibre activity – muscle fibres have a small action potential of brief duration. A motor unit consists of an anterior horn cell within the spinal cord, its axon and terminal branches, and the muscle fibres that it supplies. The number of muscle fibres innervated by each anterior horn cell varies between 10 and 200, depending on whether the muscle is used for fine or coarse control of function. There are two types of muscle fibres in humans, namely type 1 and type 2 fibres. Peripheral limb muscles contain predominantly type 2 fibres, whereas the external anal sphincter and pelvic floor muscles consist of type 1 fibres. Each motor unit potential will have the characteristic shape of electrical response. The electrical activity generated by contraction of the muscle fibres of a motor unit is recorded as the motor unit action potential. Analysis of duration and shape is of physiological value.

The striated muscles of the pelvic floor and the external anal sphincter are continuously active. Injury to the afferent nerves results in fibrillation of the muscles, which can be recorded. Investigation of the striated pelvic floor muscles has been directed at recording changes in motor unit potentials by detecting patterns which suggest muscle re-innervation.

Concentric needle EMG

Concentric needle electrodes are commonly used and consist of bare-tipped steel wire approximately 0.1 mm in diameter with an insulating resin. The area of uptake of the electrode is small and any electrical activity recorded is of the muscle into which the electrode is inserted. The recording surface is 0.5 × 0.15 mm in size at the bare tip of the wire. Individual muscle fibre action potentials cannot, however, be identified reliably using concentric needle electrodes.

The normal motor unit action potentials are biphasic (one positive, one negative peak) with a period of recovery. The mean motor unit potential duration in individuals with normal anal and urinary sphincter muscle is 5–7.5 ms.

Action potentials become polyphasic when sphincter muscle becomes denervated, and the mean motor unit potential duration is prolonged. Patients with faecal incontinence and denervation of puborectalis therefore have prolonged motor unit potential duration[16]. It also increases with age.

Technique of sphincter mapping

The patient is placed in the left lateral position. A digital examination is performed and the site of the suspected sphincter defect identified. The sweep trace is set to 100 ms/division with filter settings set at 20 Hz and 5 kHz. A concentric needle is then passed into apparently healthy muscle at the edge of the defect, and subsequently passed to map the defect until healthy muscle is identified on the opposite side of the defect. This is usually painful and the number of passes should be kept to a minimum. In some patients it may be necessary to map the whole sphincter circumference. This technique has largely been replaced by transanal ultrasonography.

Single-fibre EMG recordings

The single-fibre EMG electrode that has an uptake radius of 270 μm can record the activity of individual muscle fibres within a motor unit. The electrode consists of a needle slightly narrower than 0.1 mm, filled with resin. A central wire opens midshaft through a 25-μm gap. The cannula of the electrode represents the reference electrode and a separate ground electrode is also required. An amplifier with a 500-Hz low-frequency filter setting and a trigger delay line are required with the amplifier set at 2–5 ms/division. The mean duration of motor unit potentials consisting of more than one component recorded by this method is less than 8 ms.

To perform single-fibre EMG, right and left lateral perianal stabs are made without anaesthetic and 20 different recordings are taken from each muscle. The fibre density is assessed by counting the number of peaks in the EMG recording per stab. All action potentials greater than 100 μV are acceptable. The 20 recordings are totalled and then averaged (Figure 6.4a).

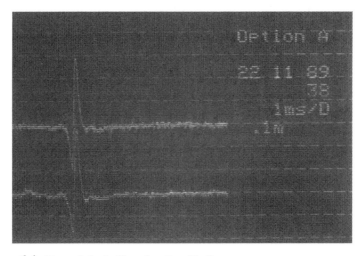

Figure 6.4a Normal single fibre density of 1-2.

After injury to the motor unit, re-innervation will result in an increase in fibre density because there will be more fibres innervated by a single axon within the uptake area. In normal individuals the fibre density of most muscles is less than two, although this increases slightly with age (Figure 6.4b).

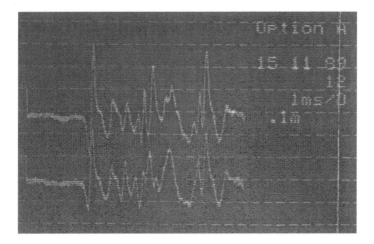

Figure 6.4b Abnormal single fibre density - one stimuli yielding activity in 11 muscle fibres.

Normal fibre density in the external sphincter muscle is 1.5 ($\pm$ 0.16). A fibre density greater than 2.0 indicates denervation and re-innervation of the muscle. Fibre density increases with age. In addition, it is increased in patients with faecal incontinence, rectal prolapse and conditions that are associated with straining at stool.

Surface EMG recordings

Anal sphincter EMG activity may be detected by surface recordings that are inserted into the anal canal (plug electrodes) or placed on perianal skin. Such EMG recordings are useful for demonstration of sphincter recruitment or inhibition while asking the patient to perform specific activities such as simulated defecation. They also enjoy the considerable additional advantage of being more comfortable for the patient compared with needle EMG[17]. The primary disadvantage of this technique is that it does not differentiate between internal and external sphincter activity.

Combined prolonged anorectal manometry with EMG recordings

One major criticism of anorectal physiology testing is that the tests are short-lived, carried out usually with the individual in the left lateral position. In addition, the embarrassment factor of perhaps being incontinent in the presence of observers/ investigators would prevent the patient from fully carrying out instructions such as attempted defecation. To overcome these 'laboratory artefacts', prolonged recording systems consisting of EMG electrodes and solid-state manometers were designed.

One example of this system is the Gaeltec 7 MPR recorder. The recorder is a digital system that possesses an events marker and a clock facility. This allows the individual being studied to mark 'events' such as defecation and micturition on the recording and make a note of the time in a diary, allowing subsequent analysis of such activities. The recorder has seven channels, allowing simultaneous EMG recordings of the internal anal sphincter, external anal sphincter and puborectalis muscle, combined with four manometric recording channels. The method uses concentric EMG electrodes inserted into the pelvic floor and anal sphincter muscles. The manometer consists of four solid-state pressure microtransducers mounted on a silicon probe 3 mm in diameter. Once inserted, the manometer will simultaneously record upper rectal, midrectal, upper anal canal and midanal canal pressures. The technique is adaptable in that it does not require a combination of EMG and manometric recordings to function. Manometry alone may therefore be performed, which is often more acceptable to the patient.

Sensation

The anus

Histological examination of the anal canal has revealed it to be profusely supplied with organized and free nerve endings extending from the anal verge to the top of the columns above the dentate line[18]. Pain, heat, cold and light touch are all sensations that are present in this area, although less precise than that of adjacent perianal skin[19]. Anal sensation is mediated via the pudendal nerves to the S2–S4 nerves. Topical application of lignocaine (lidocaine) does not impair maximum basal anal sphincter pressure, nor does it impair continence to rectally infused saline. The volume of infused saline required to produce sustained internal anal sphincter relaxation is increased and is associated with a reduction in the strength and capability of the external anal sphincter to maintain contraction. It can be concluded that normal anal sensation may not be essential for continence, although voluntary sphincter contraction depends partly on sensory input. Excision of the anal transition zone after restorative proctocolectomy does not impair continence, however, compared with patients who have not undergone mucosectomy[20].

Continent individuals do, however, have an awareness of the requirement to pass rectal contents and are then able to determine whether it is socially acceptable to do so. This awareness appears to be most acute during the sampling reflex. Various methods using different types of stimuli have been developed to assess anal sensation.

Electrical

A 14-gauge Nelaton catheter is used for this purpose by attaching two copper electrodes spaced 1 cm apart at the tip. Copper wires are connected to the electrodes and a constant-current generator. The ring electrode may be custom made but is also commercially available. The stimulator in most modern EMG machines is suitable for providing the electrical stimulus. The stimulus is set at 0.1 ms at a rate of 5 Hz in increasing strength between 1 and 25 mA. The threshold sensation, which is usually a throbbing or burning type of feeling, is measured at the lower, mid- and upper anal canal. There are no significant differences in electrosensitivity thresholds between men and nulliparous women. It is likely that anal canal and rectal electrosensitivity decline with increasing age. Acceptable normal ranges are:

- Lower anal canal: mean 4.5 (range 3.0–7.0) mA
- Midanal canal: mean 4.0 (range 2.0–6.0) mA
- Upper anal canal: mean 5.5 (range 3.0–8.0) mA.

The measurement of anal canal electrosensitivity is best carried out after measurement of the length of the anal canal so that an accurate impression may be obtained of where the electrode should be placed.

Anal sensation is increased in patients with anal fissure and blunted in patients with haemorrhoids or rectal prolapse, and those with symptoms of faecal incontinence.

Thermal

Rectal temperature is lower than that in the anal canal[21]. The anal canal mucosa is highly sensitive to temperature changes between 32°C and 42°C. The technique is somewhat complex and therefore has not found its way into routine clinical assessments. Testing for temperature discrimination involves pumping of water at three different temperatures through a probe. The temperature in the probe is rapidly changed and this can be detected by anal mucosa.

The rectum

The rectum is sensitive to distension but is insensitive to painful stimuli. The motor endings found in the anal canal mucosa are not found in the rectum. Balloon distension of the rectum produces a 'pelvic' sensation. This is likely to be mediated by pelvic floor rather than rectal mucosa nerve endings. Stretch receptors and muscle spindles have been identified within pelvic floor muscles whereas there are no organized nerve endings within the rectum. This may explain why rectal-type sensation is often preserved after surgical excision of the rectum.

Electrical

The technique used is similar to that for anal mucosal electro-sensitivity described above. A constant-current stimulus of 500 µs and 10 Hz is delivered in 0.5-mA increments. The patient will report a throbbing or buzzing sensation when the threshold of sensation is reached. The measurement is performed several times and the lowest recording is considered to be the rectal sensory threshold.

Interpretation of rectal sensation to electrical stimuli should be interpreted with some caution because there is marked circumferential sensory threshold variation. In addition, normal 'rectal' sensation can be observed in patients who have undergone rectal excision, which suggests that sensation in the pelvic floor musculature is being measured rather than that in the rectal mucosa[22].

Balloon distension

Rectal sensation can be assessed by balloon distension as described earlier in the section on rectal compliance and the rectoanal inhibitory reflex. Distension with water or air is felt at similar volumes. Patients with faecal incontinence usually have normal sensation on balloon testing. One exception is a small subgroup of patients with normal anal sphincters who exhibit abnormal rectal contractility on saline infusion or premature internal sphincter relaxation.

Data about rectal sensitivity should be interpreted with caution. Maximal tolerated volumes are not uniformly reproducible for a given individual and differ widely between individuals. The distension stimulus may be poorly defined because, with increasing distension, varying degrees of balloon elongation may occur depending on rectal wall compliance. Disturbances of rectal sensation are reflected by changes in balloon pressure, and not necessarily by changes in volume needed to provoke a given sensation. Abnormal rectal sensation as assessed by filling a rectal balloon can therefore reflect impaired viscoelastic properties of the rectal wall, rather than disturbed sensation.

Comparisons of results between different laboratories may also be difficult because of differences in technique. The distance that a catheter is inserted into the rectum and the height of the balloon in the rectum will influence rectal sensory threshold recordings. Gentle manipulation of the catheter so that the base of the balloon is consistently lying on the pelvic floor is one method of trying to correct for this. Threshold of sensation is lower with smaller incremental amounts or with slower inflation. It is also lower with intermittent inflation compared with continuous inflation with a pump. This would suggest that the sensory receptor, which triggers rectal sensation, is not a simple volume or pressure receptor but is more likely to be a slowly adapting mechanoreceptor.

Nerve stimulation techniques

Techniques of nerve stimulation provide objective assessment of neuromuscular function as well as more accurate identification of the nerve or muscle injury/lesion. Most standard EMG machines are suitable for pudendal nerve studies. Various software packages for anorectal manometry offer the added facility for recording needle EMG so that a dedicated EMG machine is not always necessary. A constant current stimulator should be used, with 20 mA (or 50 V) being the maximal stimulus. The stimulus to be delivered should be increased in small steps to avoid any sudden strong muscle contractions. Filter settings should be between 20 Hz and 5 kHz, and the sweep speed should be set at 2 ms/division.

Spinal nerve latency

The central component of motor innervation of the pelvic floor can be assessed by transcutaneous spinal stimulation. With the patient in the left lateral position, an electrode is placed vertically across the lumbar spine, usually between L1 and L4. The puborectalis or external anal sphincter response can be detected either by a surface anal plug electrode mounted on a transrectal finger glove or by an intramuscular needle electrode. The difference in latencies from L1 to L4 is known as the spinal latency ratio. This ratio is increased in patients with a proximal nerve lesion such as disc disease or spinal canal stenosis. The spinal latency ratio is also increased in patients with faecal incontinence. In the vast majority of cases this is the result of slowed conduction in the pudendal nerves. Where there is no obvious predisposing cause for incontinence, however, spinal stimulation may be used to demonstrate a cauda equina lesion. Patients with faecal incontinence where spinal stimulation may be indicated are therefore men or nulliparous women without endoanal or EMG evidence of direct sphincter injury and with no evidence of a rectal prolapse. Puborectalis is innervated directly by S3 and S4 and therefore latency measurements for this muscle can be performed only by spinal cord stimulation. Normal results are shown in Table 6.1.

Table 6.1 Normal latency measurements

	External anal sphincter	Puborectalis
L1 latency (ms)	5.5 ± 0.4	4.8 ± 0.4
L4 latency (ms)	4.4 ± 0.4	3.7 ± 0.4
Spinal latency ratio	1.33 ± 0.1	1.3 ± 0.1

Pudendal nerve terminal motor latency

Pudendal nerve stimulation is used to assess the distal motor innervation of the pelvic floor. Terminal motor latency of the pudendal nerve can be determined by a transrectal nerve stimulator. The device consists of two stimulating electrodes positioned at the tip of the index gloved finger and two recording electrodes incorporated into its base (see Figure 6.5). With the patient in the left lateral position, the electrodes on the fingertip are brought into contact with the ischial spine on each side. A square wave stimulus is delivered and the tracing is examined for evidence of external sphincter contraction as detected by the recording electrodes (see Figure 6.6). This confirms accurate localization of the pudendal

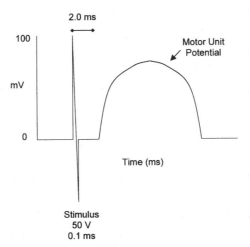

Figure 6.5 Pudendal nerve terminal motor latency: St Mark's electrode.

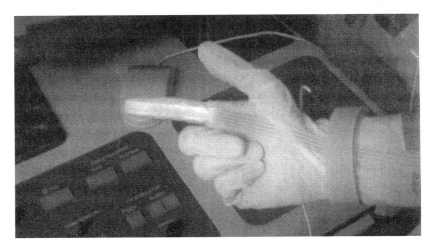

Figure 6.6 Tracing of a pudendal nerve terminal motor latency.

nerve. A stimulus of 10 mA is then delivered and the latency between the stimulus and external sphincter contraction measured. The normal pudendal nerve latency is 1.9 ± 0.2 ms. It is increased in older patients (2.1 ± 0.2 ms), and those with faecal incontinence, rectal prolapse or intractable constipation[23]. The presence of prolonged pudendal nerve latencies does not exclude a patient from operative repair of an anal sphincter defect, but it would place the patient in a category whereby long-term results may be poor because of denervation.

Assessment of rectal evacuation

Impaired evacuation commonly occurs because of a physical impediment to stool transit, e.g. tumour or stricture formation. In the absence of an organic, anatomical or extracolonic cause, 'constipation' is the result of colonic dysmotility, disordered defecation[24] or a combination of the two. The normal response to straining is silencing of electrical activity of the external anal sphincter and puborectalis, with sphincter relaxation. In patients with obstructed defecation, puborectalis may increase its activity and compound anorectal outlet obstruction[25]. In general, the following criteria define outlet obstruction:

• Demonstration of puborectalis EMG recruitment greater than 50 per cent upon straining
• Evidence of adequate rectal evacuation pressure (> 50 cmH$_2$O)
• The presence of defective evacuation (see Chapter 7).

EMG findings alone are misleading – they need to be related to balloon expulsion studies and radiological evidence of incomplete evacuation (see Chapter 7).

Rectal balloon expulsion

Rectal evacuation may be assessed by patient expulsion of an inflated balloon from the rectum. The test may be carried out with the patient in the left lateral position or sitting on a commode. A pear-shaped balloon attached to a catheter is inserted into the rectum with the patient in the left lateral position, and filled with 50 ml water. Alternatively, the balloon may be inflated to the volume of threshold rectal sensation. Slight traction may be placed on the balloon to draw it down on to the pelvic floor. Weights may be applied to the balloon, as a modification via a pulley system, up to a maximum of 200 g until the balloon is expelled. The ability to pass the balloon is not impaired by the presence or size of a coexisting rectocele, or by the presence of a rectal intussusception.

Balloon expulsion attempts to simulate defecation, which is a complex dynamic activity. The test has been criticized for being unphysiological, particularly with the patient in the left lateral position. A recent study found that both normal individuals and patients with obstructed defecation were unable to expel a rectal balloon. The test should not therefore be interpreted in isolation without EMG and radiological assessment of evacuation.

Artificial stool evacuation

Efficiency of defecation may be measured by calculating the percentage of artificial radiolabelled stool evacuated from the rectum. Normal individuals evacuate 60 ± 6 per cent of stool in 10 seconds, but this is significantly reduced in patients with obstructed defecation.

Saline continence test[27, 28]

The continence mechanism in patients with incontinence can be assessed by infusing saline at 37°C intrarectally in the presence of an anorectal manometer and EMG electrodes, and recording the volume at which the individual becomes incontinent. Normal individuals can retain volumes of up to 1500 ml saline.

Three patterns of activity have been identified to occur in normal individuals during this test, namely, rectal contractions, internal sphincter relaxation and external anal sphincter recruitment. Before complete internal sphincter relaxation and peak rectal pressure, phasic external sphincter recruitment has already begun. This is followed by more continuous external sphincter activity above basic levels as long as the rectum is distended.

Incontinent patients may demonstrate two distinct variations to the pattern seen in normal individuals. In some, rectal infusion results in normal rectal contractions and internal sphincter relaxation, but with little compensatory activity in the external anal sphincter. Such patients often show diminished anorectal sensation. It is not always clear therefore, without supplementary manometry and electrophysiology assessments, whether the external sphincter is neuropathic in these patients. A second observed pattern is a sustained early reduction in internal sphincter activity as signified in resting anal pressure. This is usually combined with irregular contractions of the external anal sphincter as demonstrated using surface electrodes. This second pattern suggests a primary dysfunction of the internal anal sphincter with perhaps a combination of dysfunction with the external anal sphincter. Once again, supplementary tests including manometry, endoanal ultrasonography and electrophysiology tests would clarify this.

References

1. Miller R, Bartolo DCC, James D et al. Air-filled microballoon manometry for use in anorectal physiology. Br J Surg 1989; 76: 72-75
2. Sun WM, Read NW, Prior A et al. Sensory and motor responses to rectal distension vary according to rate and pattern of balloon inflation. Gastroenterology 1990; 99: 1008-1015
3. Varma JS, Smith AN. Anorectal profilometry with the microtransducer. Br J Surg 1987; 71: 867-869
4. Coller JA. Clinical application of anorectal manometry. Gastroenterol Clinics North Am 1987; 16: 17-33
5. Nivatvongs S, Stern HS, Fryd DS. The length of the anal canal. Dis Colon Rectum 1981; 24: 600-601
6. Lestar B, Penninckx F, Kerremans R. The composition of anal basal pressure. An in-vivo and in-vitro study in man. Int J Colorectal Dis 1989; 4: 118-122
7. McHugh SM, Diamant NE. Anal canal pressure profile: a reappraisal as determined by rapid pullthrough technique. Gut 1987; 28: 1234-1241
8. McHugh SM, Diamant NE. Effect of age, gender and parity on anal canal pressures. Contribution of impaired anal sphincter function to faecal continence. Dig Dis Sci 1987; 32: 726-736
9. Goligher JC, Hughes ESR. Sensibility of the rectum and colon: its role in the mechanism of anal continence. Lancet 1951; i: 543-548
10. Sorenson M, Rasmussen O, Tetzscher T et al. Physiological variation in rectal compliance. Br J Surg 1992; 79: 1106-1108
11. Rao GN, Drew PJ, Monson JRT, Duthie GS. Physiology of rectal sensations. A mathematic approach. Dis Colon Rectum 1997; 40: 298-306
12. Alstrup NI, Skjoldbye B, Rasmussen O et al. Rectal compliance determined by rectal endosonography. Dis Colon Rectum 1995; 38: 32-36
13. O'Kelly TJ, Brading AF, Mortensen NJ. Nerve mediated relaxation of the human internal anal sphincter. Gut 1993; 34: 689-693
14. Broens PMA, Penninckx FM, Lestar B et al. The trigger for rectal filling sensation. Int J Colorectal Dis 1994; 9: 1-4
15. Percy JP, Neill ME, Swash M, Parks AG. Electrophysiological study of the pelvic floor. Lancet 1981; i: 16-17
16. Kiff ES, Barnes P, Swash M. Evidence of pudendal neuropathy in patients with perineal descent and chronic straining at stool. Gut 1984; 25: 1279-1282
17. Jost WH, Ecker KW, Schimrigk K. Surface versus needle electrodes in determination of motor conduction time to the external anal sphincter. Int J Colorectal Dis 1994; 9: 197-199
18. Duthie HL, Gairns FN. Sensory nerve endings and sensation in the anal region of man. Br J Surg 1960; 47: 585-595
19. Read MG, Read NW. The role of anorectal sensation in preserving continence. Gut 1982; 23: 345-347

20. Keighley MRB, Winslet MC, Yoshioka K et al. Discrimination is not impaired by excision of the anal transitional zone after restorative proctocolectomy. Br J Surg 1987; 74: 1118-1121
21. Miller R, Bartolo DCC, Cervero C et al. Anorectal temperature sensation: a comparison of normal and incontinent patients. Br J Surg 1987; 74: 511-515
22. Meagher AP, Kennedy ML, Lubowski DZ. Rectal mucosal electrosensitivity - what is being tested? Int J Colorectal Dis 1996; 11: 29-33
23. Kiff ES, Swash M. Slowed conduction in the pudendal nerves in idiopathic (neurogenic) faecal incontinence. Br J Surg 1984; 71: 614-616
24. Preston DM, Lennard-Jones JE. Anismus in chronic constipation. Dig Dis Sci 1985; 30: 413-418
25. Fleshman JW, Dreznick Z, Cohen E et al. Balloon expulsion test facilitates diagnosis of pelvic floor outlet obstruction due to nonrelaxing puborectalis muscle. Dis Colon Rectum 1992; 35: 1019-1025
26. Barnes PRH, Lennard-Jones JE. Balloon expulsion from the rectum in constipation of different types. Gut 1985; 26: 1049-1052
27. Read NW, Haynes WG, Bartolo DCC et al. Use of anorectal manometry during rectal infusion of saline to investigate sphincter function in incontinent patients. Gastroenterology 1983; 85: 105-113
28. Bartolo DCC, Read MG, Read NW. The saline continence test. Dynamic studies in faecal incontinence, haemorrhoids and the descending perineum syndrome. Acta Gastroenterol Belg 1985; 48: 39-50

Chapter 7
Functional radiology of the gastrointestinal tract

GED R AVERY

Functional gastrointestinal imaging is becoming increasingly popular in the assessment of both gastrointestinal transit and defecation. As with all radiological investigations, it is important that the radiologist has a good understanding of the clinical problem, and that the clinician has a good understanding of the information that can be provided by the examination requested.

The mainstays of investigation are radiographic and nuclear medicine studies, although more recently both ultrasonography and magnetic resonance imaging (MRI) have been used.

Radiographic techniques provide good spatial resolution and are the methods of choice for assessing structural lesions or mucosal detail. However, the transit studies have to be performed with non-physiological materials: either barium or radio-opaque markers. Prolonged screening times can lead to high radiation exposure for the patient and the interpretation is often subjective.

Nuclear medicine techniques allow the use of physiological materials tagged with a radioactive tracer. The patient's radiation exposure is independent of the time taken to acquire the data, which can be quantitatively assessed. However, the spatial resolution is poor and this can be troublesome, such as in differentiating terminal ileum and caecum.

Transit studies can be divided into oesophageal, gastric, small bowel and colonic studies. The methods used vary for each region; these are discussed and comparison made between the available techniques. It is important to be aware of the normal physiology when interpreting the results, and a brief description of normal motility is given.

Defecating proctography is used to assess disturbance in normal anorectal function, including obstructed defecation and constipation. Structural abnormalities including rectocele and mucosal prolapse can be demonstrated. Techniques and interpretation are also discussed.

Oesophageal transit

Oesophageal transit is initiated by pharyngeal activity; a primary peristaltic wave moves down the oesophagus at 2-5 cm/s reaching the distal oesophagus 4-10 seconds later. Distension of the distal oesophagus may trigger a further peristaltic wave. The lower oesophageal sphincter relaxes for up to 4 seconds with an after-contraction to clear the remaining food into the stomach.

If a second oral swallow occurs before this sequence is complete, it can disrupt the primary peristaltic wave and lead to poor emptying of the mid-oesophagus[1].

Patient preparation is important; patients should be starved for 3-4 hours before to ensure that the stomach is empty, and asked not to smoke during this time because this may disturb oesophageal motility. The patient's drug history should be reviewed; agents that may increase peristaltic activity include benzodiazepines, β-adrenergic drugs and metoclopramide. Reduced peristalsis can occur with calcium antagonists and glucagon – this may be used in barium studies for structural abnormalities.

Radiographic techniques

The barium swallow is a routine investigation in the management of dysphagia and is a sensitive examination for structural abnormalities. Smooth muscle relaxants, e.g. glucagon or hyoscine butylbromide (Buscopan), may be used to aid evaluation of structural lesions.

Videofluoroscopy is the mainstay of oesophageal motility investigation; in this, swallowing is recorded on video rather than static images. A high-quality video recorder is needed to allow good slow-motion and frame-by-frame display.

Liquid barium is the most common agent, although barium-impregnated marshmallows, bread or biscuits can be used to assess the transit of solid food. If there is concern about aspiration, it is possible to use water-soluble contrast of low osmolarity; this medium should also be used if an oesophageal perforation or leak is suspected.

The examination starts with the patient erect. A bolus of contrast is swallowed in a single gulp and the patient is then asked to keep his or her mouth open to reduce secondary swallowing. Further swallows are performed with the patient prone or prone oblique; this minimizes the effect of gravity on the oesophageal transit. A minimum of four swallows are usually performed. The swallows are recorded on a video and reviewed.

The primary peristaltic wave is visible as an inverted V passing distally, stripping the barium down the oesophagus; occasionally proximal escape of barium can occur at the level of the aortic arch. In the absence of other altered motility this can be a normal variant, particularly in elderly people[2]. Secondary peristaltic waves occur with local oesophageal distension and progress distally. Tertiary contractions are non-peristaltic and of variable strength, and may be multiple; these are associated with motility disorders but are also a response to structural abnormalities or gastro-oesophageal reflux. However, they are also common in elderly people, in which group they need to be correlated with clinical symptoms[2]. Oesophageal distension and lower oesophageal sphincter (LOS) function are also assessed.

If there is concern about a dysfunctional pharyngeal phase of swallowing, it is of value to perform the examination with a speech and language therapist present so that modifications to swallowing techniques can be assessed.

Nuclear medicine techniques

Scintigraphic techniques of monitoring oesophageal transit are not as widely used as videofluoroscopy. Its advantages are the ability to quantify bolus transport and the low patient dose allowing multiple swallows or repeat studies; the main disadvantage is poor spatial resolution.

The preferred radionuclide is technetium-99m (^{99m}Tc). This is readily available with a radioactive half-life ($t_{1/2}$) of 6 hours; it emits a photon of 140 keV which is ideal for imaging with a gamma camera. It can be incorporated into a variety of radiopharmaceuticals, which can then be used to label different foods and liquids. Other agents have been used, e.g. krypton-81m (^{81m}Kr). This is a very short-lived radioactive gas, with a $t_{1/2}$ of 13 seconds, which can be dissolved in water, its rapid clearance of activity allowing multiple studies in quick succession.

Patient preparation is again important and, as previously stated, is as for radiographic studies. The most common positions used are erect and supine; it can be helpful to perform the examination in both positions – supine examinations may reveal more abnormalities but erect examinations may help differentiate scleroderma from achalasia[3].

The patient is asked to swallow either liquids (labelled water or fruit juice) or solids (labelled scrambled egg/omelette often being used).

A rapid acquisition of 1–3 frames with an image matrix of 64 × 64 pixels is generally used. This illustrates one of the major problems with nuclear medicine – poor spatial resolution. (For digital fluoroscopy the image matrix can be up to 2000 × 2000 pixels.) However, it is possible to review the data either qualitatively with cine-reviews or quantitatively by measuring count rates within the oesophagus. Transit times and clearances times can be calculated for either the whole oesophagus or the proximal, mid- and distal oesophagus separately.

Clinical indications

There are several groups of patients who may suffer from oesophageal motility disorder, including:

- Patients with dysphagia and normal endoscopy
- Patients with non-cardiac central chest pain
- Patients with known scleroderma.

Common motility problems that can be detected with videofluoroscopy include diffuse oesophageal spasm and non-specific oesophageal motility disorders, both of which demonstrate tertiary contractions, although in the former the LOS functions normally. In achalasia, absent primary peristalsis and absent or incomplete opening of the LOS with or without oesophageal dilatation is reliably demonstrated[4].

Motility disorders can also be seen with connective tissue disorders, particularly scleroderma; poor distal oesophageal peristalsis, an incompetent LOS and gastro-oesophageal reflux are commonly demonstrated[4].

Nuclear medicine has a minor role to play, although it can demonstrate the same signs as videofluoroscopy. One of its main advantages is in assessing the effects of treatment with quantitative data.

Gastric transit

Gastric motility is regulated by the different motor functions of the proximal stomach (fundus and upper third of the body) and the distal stomach. The proximal stomach relaxes during feeding, to allow a constant pressure to be maintained within the stomach and the proximal stomach to act as a reservoir. This is followed by a slow tonic contraction, which increases the intragastric pressure, propelling food into the distal stomach. The differential pressure between the stomach and the duodenum is the major regulator in liquid transit, which is therefore dependent on proximal stomach function.

In the distal stomach, peristaltic contractions occur at a rate of 3/min to convert the food into chyme, which is then allowed to pass through the pylorus. Larger indigestible solid particles are retained within the stomach as a result of synchronous closure of the pylorus with the antral contraction. Stomach emptying is dependent on the carbohydrate/fat content and the acidity of the chyme. These are monitored by receptors within the duodenum which feed back to control antral contractions and pyloric pressure. Carbohydrates empty quicker than fats, and acidity reduces the rate of emptying. The indigestible particles are eventually cleared during the fasting state when contractile activity is accompanied by pyloric opening.

It is important to remember this regulation of gastric emptying when evaluating the results of solid phase emptying studies; the transit times obtained will be dependent on the nature of the test meal.

The emptying of liquids from the stomach is usually mono-exponential whereas solid food emptying has an initial lag phase, then a period with a constant emptying rate and a further, much slower phase when the stomach is almost empty.

Patient preparation is again important; some drugs may affect gastric emptying and, as for oesophageal motility, should be stopped for 48 hours before the test and the patient starved overnight. If the patient has diabetes he or she should take the usual morning insulin just before the test meal because hypoglycaemia may delay gastric emptying[5].

In contradistinction to the oesophagus, radiographic studies are less well accepted than radionuclide imaging. Newer techniques that have been used include both ultrasonography and MRI.

Radiographic techniques

Barium studies are useful for assessing the anatomy of the stomach, but it is a non-physiological material that may influence gastric emptying[5].

Radio-opaque markers have been studied; these are indigestible solid particles that will remain in the stomach until fasting state contractions allow their clearance. They have been used to assess gastroparesis, with films taken at 2-hourly intervals after ingestion for up to 6 hours (all markers are normally cleared by this time), with the results showing good correlation with symptoms in patients suspected of gastroparesis[6].

Nuclear medicine techniques

It is important that a standardized technique is used – gastric emptying is affected by the content of the meal and patient positioning. Solid emptying requires a radiopharmaceutical with good labelling efficiency and high stability; this is provided by ^{99m}Tc-sulphur colloid which binds to egg (usually given as scrambled egg) or liver. The emptying rates of these two agents are different, being slower for labelled liver, which most closely resembles indigestible solid particle emptying. Liquid emptying can be assessed either before solid emptying with [^{99m}Tc]pertechnetate-labelled water or simultaneously using ^{111}In-DTPA-labelled water (water labelled with indium-111-diethylenetriaminepenta-acetic acid), the gamma-camera being able to distinguish between the emitted γ radiation of these two radionuclides.

The examination is usually performed with the patient erect or semi-recumbent in an attempt to separate the stomach from small intestine activity; if the patient is supine, emptying is significantly slower[7]. Acquisitions usually last up to 2 hours at a rate of 1 frame/minute, although longer acquisitions may be required if emptying is slow.

For quantification of the data, two corrections to the observed count rates need to be considered – decay and attenuation corrections. Significant decay of ^{99m}Tc occurs over a 2-hour acquisition as a result of its short $t_{1/2}$ of 6 hours, and the count rates should be routinely corrected to allow for this.

Attenuation correction is required as a result of the shape of the stomach, because activity moves from the posterior fundus to the anteriorly placed antrum. The distance of the activity from the camera alters, varying the count rate in the absence of gastric emptying. A dual-headed camera, with the heads positioned anteriorly and posteriorly, allows a geometric mean count rate to be obtained. If a single-headed camera is used, frequent anterior and posterior views can be obtained, although patient disturbance may affect gastric emptying.

The resultant data can be used to express gastric emptying in several ways. The simplest is to report the time to 50 per cent emptying $(t_{1/2})$. This is suitable for liquid emptying, although it does not address the lag phase in solid emptying, and other methods have been used for this, including power – exponential functions[7].

The normal ranges of $t_{1/2}$ vary between investigators as a result of differences in technique, and therefore each centre should determine its own normal range. Quoted ranges for the $t_{1/2}$ solid meal vary between 28–40 minutes and 78–160 minutes[6, 8]. Recent studies have also detected gender-related differences in gastric emptying with slower emptying of solid meals in women compared with men[9].

It is also possible to measure the frequency and amplitude of antral contractions by acquiring 1-second frames over a 4-minute period; this can be used to identify the alterations in motility causing delayed gastric emptying[10].

Ultrasonography

This can be used to assess two parameters: motility of the distal stomach wall by visualizing peristaltic contractions, and gastric emptying of liquids by serial measurement of the antral cross-sectional area[11]. It is a non-invasive technique with no radiation. However, it is operator dependent and it is difficult to assess proximal gastric function or solid emptying[5]. It is not currently a commonly used technique.

Magnetic resonance imaging

This is a radiation-free, non-invasive technique. Recent advances in MRI technology allow assessment of gastric motility with frame acquisitions every 1–2 seconds giving good temporal resolution. Gastric volumes can also be calculated and corrected for gastric secretions by exploiting the differences in signal characteristics between these and the test meal; emptying rates can therefore be calculated[12].

It is a time-consuming technique that can take up to 2 hours' scanning time[12] – a major disadvantage given the heavy clinical demand for MRI. Currently, this technique remains a research tool.

Clinical indications

Gastric emptying studies are useful in the following groups:

- Patients suspected of gastroparesis, in particular diabetic gastroparesis
- Patients with symptoms following gastric surgery
- Patients with non-ulcer dyspepsia.

Gastroparesis is often demonstrated on solid phase emptying because normal liquid emptying can be maintained despite severe gastroparesis for solids. Delayed gastric emptying can occur in up to 50 per cent of patients with type 1 diabetes but this must be correlated with patient symptoms[5].

After gastric surgery either symptomatic rapid gastric emptying ('dumping') or gastric stasis can occur. Stasis can be present despite a widely patent anastomosis.

Delayed gastric emptying has been reported in up to 80 per cent of patients with non-ulcer dyspepsia; demonstration of this may be helpful, because this group may respond to prokinetic agents[13].

Small bowel transit

Small bowel motility varies between the fasting and postprandial states; it also alters between the proximal small bowel and the ileum. The migrating motor complex (MMC) occurs in the fasting state and is characterized by three phases. Phase 3 is the most distinctive and is a succession of contractions occurring approximately 11 times/min and lasting for about 5 min; these usually start at the ligament of Treitz, migrate through the small bowel and terminate in the ileum. This phase recurs at 90- to 110-min intervals, in between which is a period of minimal peristalsis (phase 1) followed by irregular contractions (phase 2).

Food intake initiates irregular contractions, the duration of which depends on vagal control and caloric content of the meal – the higher the content the longer the duration of activity[14]. These distinctions are less clear in the ileum, which also responds to caecal reflux by prolonged propulsive contractions.

Radiographic techniques

Barium is rarely used to assess small bowel transit. It is, however, useful in the diagnosis of obstruction although, in subacute/partial small bowel obstruction, false-negative studies can occur. Recently radio-opaque markers have been used to evaluate suspected subacute obstruction not demonstrated on barium studies. They may coalesce in the region of partial obstruction as a result of variations between liquid and solid motility[15].

Nuclear medicine techniques

As with assessment of motility elsewhere within the gut, there is no standard method for assessing small bowel transit. ^{99m}Tc and ^{111}In can both be used as a solid meal (^{99m}Tc-sulphur colloid with egg), liquid ^{111}In-DTPA-labelled water or ^{111}In attached to resin pellets.

Acquisition protocols vary. It is a time-consuming test lasting several hours and therefore dependent on the workload of the department; it is undertaken as either a continuous acquisition or multiple images at 10- to 30-min intervals.

There are difficulties in accurately quantifying small bowel transit as a result of two problems: the need to compensate for gastric emptying and the poor spatial resolution impeding differentiation of the caecum from the terminal ileum.

The simplest method of measuring small bowel transit is to time the initial arrival of activity within the caecum of orally administered activity. Limited spatial resolution may be a problem and tracer has been shown to accumulate in the terminal ileum before entering the caecum. This is an easier site to define and the rate of accumulation of activity in the distal small bowel can be used as an index of small bowel motility[16].

Other methods include subtracting the time for 10 per cent gastric emptying from 10 per cent colonic filling or using mathematical deconvolution techniques. Mean transit times of approximately 160 min were obtained[17].

Clinical indications

The main use is in the evaluation of patients with constipation. It is important to distinguish patients with slow colonic transit and normal upper gastrointestinal motility from those with associated gastric/small bowel dysmotility. This latter group may have symptoms of bloating, abdominal pain and vomiting, which would not be corrected by colectomy. Colectomy should be performed only if the transit abnormality is limited to the colon[17].

Colonic transit

Colonic filling occurs mainly as a series of boluses from the terminal ileum following a meal; during fasting the filling is erratic. Two major types of colonic contraction occur – propagating and non-propagating. Propagating sequences are most prevalent in the caecum and ascending colon; most terminate close to the splenic flexure. In the distal colon, non-propagating sequences are more common and are the predominant overall colonic pattern. Occasionally, high-amplitude propagating contractions can pass along the whole length of the colon; the frequency of these varies between 4 and 10 a day[18].

Before the assessment of colonic transit, all laxatives and drugs that may affect the colon must be stopped 2 days before and for the duration of the study.

Radiographic techniques

These use radio-opaque markers within a gelatine capsule. The initial study used daily abdominal radiographs and stool radiographs to assess the transit of 20 markers. In a group of normal volunteers, at least 80 per cent of the markers were passed within 5 days[19].

A simplified approach is to give the markers on day 0, take a single radiograph on day 5 and count the residual markers. This does not assess segmental colonic transit, and further techniques have evolved to study this without the need for daily radiographs.

Three sets of distinctive markers are taken on 3 successive days and a single radiograph taken on day 4. Localization of the markers is by either gaseous outlines or bony landmarks. Using this technique, it is possible to assess transit times for the right colon, left colon and rectosigmoid. The normal ranges obtained with this technique were total colon 35 (2.1) h (mean [standard error or SE], respectively), right colon 11.3 (1.1) h, left colon 11.4 (1.4) h and rectosigmoid 12.4 (1.1) h [20].

Nuclear medicine techniques

^{111}In-DTPA is the most common agent used; it has a long $t_{1/2}$ of 2.83 days, which reduces the effect of decay on count rates and is not absorbed from the bowel. The radionuclide can be given either in a liquid or within a capsule, the coating of which is designed to dissolve in the ileocaecal area to deliver the radioactivity as a bolus to the colon [21, 22].

Imaging needs to be performed over a period of 3 days; several different acquisition protocols have been used but a comparison of two methods showed that images at 8–10 h on day 1, 24 h and 48 h allowed assessment of five patterns of colonic transit: normal, rapid, right-sided delay, left-sided delay or generalized delay [21]. To determine segmental transit, the colon is divided into at least three segments: right, left and rectosigmoid. Anterior and posterior images are obtained to give a geometric mean and therefore a count rate independent of the depth of the activity within the abdomen.

Transit times obtained with radionuclides have been shown to be comparable to radiographic techniques [23].

Clinical indications

Constipation is a common clinical problem that can be defined symptomatically as difficulty in defecation or low bowel frequency. The initial consideration is the exclusion of an obstructing lesion; a barium enema or colonoscopy is required for detection of structural lesions. Other causes include impaired motility or disorders of rectal evacuation. A combination of colonic transit studies and proctography is helpful to distinguish between these two groups of patients.

If colon transit is normal in a patient with symptoms of constipation, this may be the result of an irritable bowel syndrome [24]. Patients with prolonged colonic transit may be candidates for surgical resection which could be either partial left-sided or subtotal colectomy [25, 26]. Normal transit through the right and left colon, but delay in the rectosigmoid, is often associated with anorectal dysfunction [25].

Defecating proctography

This technique is used to evaluate dynamic changes in the anorectum and pelvic floor during defecation. Essentially, it is performed with the patient sitting on a commode and recording the evacuation of barium by videofluoroscopy.

It must be recognized that this procedure can cause significant embarrassment to the patient. It is essential to discuss the procedure with the patient, ideally before entering the examination room. The procedure should be performed in as private an environment as possible; locking the doors and the use of screens may be helpful. The number of staff present should be kept to a minimum.

Patient preparation is not necessary[27], although some centres use phosphate enemas immediately before the study[11].

Radiographic techniques

It is important to have a high-quality video recorder capable of slow motion review and a good freeze-frame facility. Care has to be taken over the design of the commode to obtain a uniform attenuation of the X-ray beam when the patient is seated, otherwise the image quality is degraded.

Thick barium paste is usually used, which can be commercially obtained[27, 28] or prepared as a mixture of barium and starch within the department[29]. Volumes of between 120 and 250 ml are administered with the patient in the left lateral decubitus position. With the patient in this position and/or sitting on the commode, radiographs are taken at rest, squeezing the pelvic floor and straining. The patient is asked to evacuate the barium while sitting on the commode and the procedure recorded on videotape.

Nuclear medicine techniques

It is possible to study anorectal function with radionuclides – labelled potato starch has been used[20]. The technique is similar to that for radiographic studies; the patient can, however, be in a separate room to the operator, and the commode design is not as important. There is a lower radiation dose to the patient, and emptying can be quantified. However, resolution is poor and pelvic landmarks not visible.

Technique variations

Contrast is often used to outline the vagina and the small bowel. Vaginal contrast can be obtained by using a tampon soaked in iodinated contrast medium. However, this may act as a splint to the posterior vaginal wall; alternative methods include using a gauze swab to introduce barium paste or mixing the paste with an aqueous gel. Small bowel contrast is obtained by the use of oral barium taken 1–1.5 h previously. These two modifications are used in particular to detect the presence of enteroceles.

Less commonly the bladder is catheterized and water-soluble iodine contrast introduced[30]. This technique allows the assessment of cystoceles, the urethral sphincter and the mobility of the urethrovesical junction.

Peritoneography is a recent addition. An anterior abdominal wall puncture is performed and 20–60 ml of non-ionic contrast medium injected into the peritoneal cavity[31]; there is visualization of the pelvic peritoneal sac during defecation and the detection of peritoneoceles.

Analysis

There are three commonly used measurements that can be made from the radiographs.

The anorectal angle (Table 7.1)

This is the angle between a line drawn along the axis of the anal canal and a line drawn along the posterior wall of the rectum.

This angle is produced by the effect of the puborectalis muscles, the impression of which can be seen on the distal posterior rectal wall. In a normal individual, contraction of the pelvic floor will decrease the angle and straining will increase it.

Table 7.1 Measurements of anorectal angles in normal volunteers[32] and asymptomatic individuals[33]

	Anorectal angle (°) on		
	Rest	Squeeze	Strain
Mean (range) in normal volunteers[32]			
Men	96 (64–125)	80 (45–116)	98 (67–123)
Women	95 (70–134)	71 (54–95)	103 (75–128)
Mean (SD) in asymptomatic individuals[33]			
Men	104 (25)	81 (23)	122 (22)
Women	112 (23)	86 (20)	129 (11)

The position of the anorectal junction

This has been described as either the point at which the parallel walls of the anal canal convert to the diverging walls of the rectum[32], or the point at which the lines of the anorectal angle intersect[33]. It is used to assess pelvic floor movement and must therefore be assessed against a static reference point. There are two options: the coccyx[33] or the inferior margin of the ischial tuberosities[32].

A position of the anorectal angle 4 cm or more below the level of coccyx at rest and/or descent of more than 4 cm during straining is considered abnormal[33]. This is known as the descending perineum syndrome and can be associated with perineal discomfort.

The width of the anal canal

This should not be measurable at rest or on squeezing the pelvic floor.

Anismus is a functional disorder of defecation, causing impaired rectal evacuation. There is a failure of the pelvic floor to relax with sustained contraction during attempts to defecate. Proctography demonstrates a delay in the initiation of defecation with prolonged evacuation time and poor rectal emptying[34]. The presence of a persisting puborectalis impression and minimal alteration in the anorectal angle during defecation have been described[35], although they are not constant features[34].

Structural disorders are commonly seen. Intussusception of the rectal wall can vary from minimal unfolding of one wall to circumferential invagination of the wall into the lumen, which progresses down the rectum during defecation. A rectal prolapse occurs when the intussusception passes through the anal canal, so that the rectal mucosa is visualized externally.

A rectocele is the herniation of the anterior wall of the rectum into the vagina and is characterized by a bulge occurring outside the line of the anterior rectal wall on defecation. Trapping of faeces can occur with the rectocele causing a feeling of incomplete evacuation, which may lead to increased straining with later development of rectal intussusception and increased perineal descent[36].

Solitary rectal ulcer is associated with a history of defecation disorders, predominantly excessive straining. The most common proctographic finding is rectal intussusception, which is thought to cause mechanical injury to the mucosa; other findings have included dysfunction of the puborectalis[37].

In the assessment of any radiological technique, it is important to be aware of the appearances in a normal population. Two studies using normal volunteers with no history of bowel disturbance demonstrated a high incidence of rectoceles of 80–100 per cent in the women and 13–40 per cent in the men[32, 38]. Although these were mainly small, between 1 and 2 cm in depth, occasional larger rectoceles with trapping of barium were noted. It was also common to see a small intrarectal intussusception, which did not interfere with emptying.

It is therefore important that the findings on defecating proctography are considered not in isolation but as part of a comprehensive assessment of rectal and pelvic floor function.

References

1. Ask P, Tibbing L. Effect of time interval between swallows on oesophageal peristalsis. Am J Physiol 1980; 238: 485–490
2. Low VHS, Rubesin SE. Contrast evaluation of the pharynx and oesophagus. Radiol Clinics North Am 1993; 31: 1265–1291
3. Parkman HP, Miller MA, Fisher RS. Role of nuclear medicine in evaluating patients with suspected gastrointestinal motility disorders. Semin Nucl Med 1995; 25: 289–305
4. Schima W, Ryan JM, Harisinghani M et al. Radiographic detection of achalasia. Diagnostic accuracy of videofluoroscopy. Clin Radiol 1998; 53: 372–375
5. Parkman HP, Harris AD, Krevsky MD et al. Gastroduodenal motility and dysmotility. An update on techniques available for evaluation. Am J Gastroenterol 1995; 90: 869–892
6. Poitras P, Pickard M, Dery R et al. Evaluation of gastric emptying function in clinical practice. Dig Dis Sci 1997; 42: 2183–2189
7. Maurer AH, Fisher RS. Current applicability of scintigraphic methods in gastroenterology. Baillière's Clin Gastroenterol 1995; 9: 71–79
8. Harding K, Robinson PJA. Gastric emptying. In: Clinicians' Guide to Nuclear Medicine, Gastroenterology. Edinburgh: Churchill Livingstone, 1991
9. Bennink R, Peeters M, Van den Maegdenbergh V et al. Comparison of total and compartmental gastric emptying and antral motility between healthy men and women. Eur J Nucl Med 1998; 25: 1293–1299
10. Urbain JL, Charles ND. Recent advances in gastric emptying scintigraphy. Semin Nucl Med 1995; 25: 318–325
11. Hveem K, Jones KL, Chatterton BE et al. Scintigraphic measurement of gastric emptying and ultrasonographic assessment of antral area. Relation to appetite. Gut 1996; 38: 816–821
12. Kunz P, Crelier GR, Schwizer W et al. Gastric emptying and motility. Assessment with MR imaging - preliminary observations. Radiology 1998; 207: 33–40
13. Jian R, Ducrot F, Ruskone A et al. Symptomatic, radionuclide and therapeutic assessment of chronic idiopathic dyspepsia. Dig Dis Sci 1989; 34: 657–664

14. Husebye E. Clinical physiology of the small bowel. In: Phillips SF, Wingate DL (eds), Functional Disorders of the Gut. Edinburgh: Churchill Livingstone, 1998

15. Johnson PA, Miner PB, Geir D et al. Value of radio-opaque markers in identifying partial small bowel obstruction. Gastroenterology 1996; 110: 1958–1963

16. Krevsky B, Maurer AH, Niewionowski T et al. The effect of verapamil on human intestinal transit. Dig Dis Sci 1992; 37: 919–924

17. Maurer AH, Krevsky B. Whole gut transit scintigraphy in the evaluation of small bowel and colon transit disorders. Semin Nucl Med 1995; 25: 326–338

18. Cook IJ. Colon and anorectum: constipation, urgency, pain syndromes. Clinical physiology. In: Phillips SF, Wingate DL (eds), Functional Disorders of the Gut. Edinburgh: Churchill Livingstone, 1998

19. Hinton JM, Lennard-Jones JE, Young AC. A new method for studying gut transit times using radio-opaque markers. Gut 1969; 10: 842–847

20. Metcalf AM, Phillips SF, Zinsmeister et al. Simplified assessment of segmental colonic transit. Gastroenterology 1987; 92: 40–47

21. Notgti A, Hutchinson R, Kumar D et al. Simplified method for the measurement of segmental colonic transit time. Gut 1994; 35: 976–981

22. Roberts JP, Newell MS, Deekes JJ et al. Oral ^{111}In-DTPA scintigraphic assessment of colonic transit in constipated subjects. Dig Dis Sci 1993; 38: 1032–1039

23. Van der Sijp JRM, Kamm MA, Nightingale JMD et al. Radioisotope determination of regional colonic transit in severe constipation: compression with radio-opaque markers. Gut 1993; 34: 402–408

24. Bouchoucha M, Devroede G, Renard P. Compartmental analysis of colonic transit reveals abnormalities in constipated patients with normal transit. Clin Sci 1995; 89: 129–135

25. De Graff EJR, Gilberts EC, Schouten WR. Role of segmental colonic transit time studies to select patients with slow transit constipation for partial left sided or subtotal colectomy. Br J Surg 1996; 83: 648–651

26. Nyam DC, Pemberton VH, Ilstrup MS et al. Long-term results of surgery for chronic constipation. Dis Colon Rectum 1997; 40: 273–279

27. Turnbull GK, Bartram CL, Lennard Jones JE. Radiologic studies of rectal evacuation in adults with idiopathic constipation. Dis Colon Rectum 1988; 31: 190–197

28. Jarge JM, Ger GC, Gonzalez L et al. Patient position during cinedefecography influence on perineal descent and other measurements. Dis Colon Rectum 1994; 37: 927–931

29. Klauser AG, Ting KH, Mangel E. Interobserver agreement in defecography. Dis Colon Rectum 1994; 37: 1310–1316

30. Altringer WE, Saclavides TJ, Dominguez JM et al. Four-contrast defecography. Pelvic 'floor-oscopy'. Dis Colon Rectum 1995; 38: 695–699

31. Bremmer S, Mellgren A, Homstrom B et al. Peritoneocele. Visualisation with defecography and peritoneography performed simultaneously. Radiology 1997; 202: 373–377

32. Shorron P, McHugh S, Diamant N et al. Defecography in normal volunteers: results and implication. Gut 1989; 30: 1737–1749

33. Goei R, Van Engelshoven J, Schouten H. Anorectal function: defecographic measurement in asymptomatic subjects. Radiology 1989; 173: 137–141

34. Halligan S, Bartram CL, Park HJ, Kamm MA. Proctographic features of anismus. Radiology 1985; 197: 679–682

35. Jorge JMN, Wexner SD, Ger GC et al. Cinedefecography and electromyography in the diagnosis of non relaxing puborectalis syndrome. Dis Colon Rectum 1993; 36: 668-676

36. Van Dam JH, Ginai AZ, Gosselink MJ et al. Role of defecography in predicting clinical outcome of rectocele repair. Dis Colon Rectum 1997; 40: 201-207

37. Guei R, Baeten C, Arends J. Solitary rectal ulcer syndrome: findings at barium enema study and defecography. Radiology 1988; 168: 303-366

38. Ikenberry S, Lappas JC, Hana MP et al. Defecography in healthy subjects: comparison of three contrast media. Radiology 1996; 201: 233-238

Chapter 8
Anorectal ultrasonography

Angela Gardiner and Geetinder Kaur

The use of endoluminal ultrasonography (ELUS) has rapidly become one of the gold standard techniques for the imaging of the anorectum over recent years. The low rectum, anal sphincters and pelvic floor in patients with a variety of anorectal diseases can be clearly visualized using the technique.

The early descriptions made of the technique were by Reid and Wild of the University of Minnesota in the early 1950s. There were no more reports made of its use again until the 1980s, at which point it was enthusiastically pursued for staging of rectal cancers. Further development over the last 15–20 years has resulted in it becoming an essential assessment tool for the evaluation of the anatomy of the rectum, anal sphincters and pelvic floor. There are a variety of indications for anorectal ultrasonography which are discussed below:

- Traumatic and idiopathic incontinence
- Perianal fistulae/abscesses
- Anal and rectal malignancy staging
- Anal sphincter assessment before surgery for anal fissure.

As the technique becomes more routinely used, it is recognized that it is not always possible for a surgeon or physician to be available to perform the investigation. With the introduction of nurse practitioners and clinical physiologists in colorectal units, it is becoming commonplace for such professionals to perform ELUS, provided that a suitable training regimen, similar to that followed for flexible sigmoidoscopy and upper gastrointestinal (GI) endoscopy, is followed. A study was performed within Castle Hill Hospital to evaluate the suitability of technical staff to perform and interpret the images obtained. Images were blindly assessed by a surgeon who was regarded as a specialist in the area; they were then passed to the physiologist and a registrar within the unit. The interpretation made by the surgeon was taken as the standard for comparison. Results showed that there was a very good correlation among the three parties and there was no reason why suitably trained technical personnel should not perform the investigation, provided that an adequate level of competence was achieved.

Equipment

The procedure can be performed in any standard patient examination room, or in the operating theatre if required. A number of manufacturers produce scanning heads suitable for endoluminal scanning. The standard equipment in most laboratories is the Bruel and Kjaer range of ultrasound scanning systems (Figure 8.1).

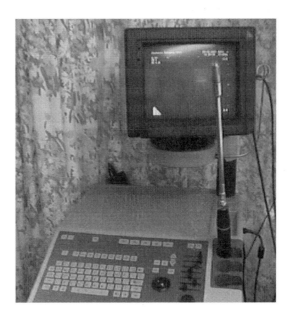

Figure 8.1 Standard ultrasound equipment for the assessment of endoluminal ultrasound.

This system consists of a 360°, rotating, hand-held probe, which is connected to the ultrasound unit; the image obtained is in the form of a complete cross-section. This type of system appears to be one of the most popular. Multifunctional transducers are available, although the 10-MHz transducer yields the highest resolution of the anal canal structure, as a result of its focal zone being between 1

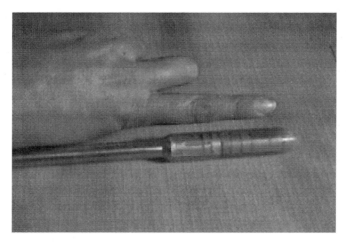

Figure 8.2 Hand plastic cone covering transducer head shown in relation to index finger.

and 4 cm. The transducer is covered with a hard protective plastic cone which slightly distends the anal canal (Figure 8.2).

Generally, there is no requirement for bowel preparation before the study in the laboratory setting. However, if further studies are to be performed, such as manometry, it may be appropriate to administer a glycerin suppository before the investigations. If manometry is necessary, it is best practice for the ultrasonogram to be carried out at the end of the investigations because this may cause a distortion to the anal canal, which may affect the manometric results. The full examination takes around 10–15 minutes to complete and is only minimally uncomfortable for the patient; the only exception to this is patients with a painful anal fissure. In these circumstances, the technique may be completed under an anaesthetic in the operating theatre, or local anaesthetic gel may be applied to the anal canal.

The hard plastic cone must be purged of all air, because air bubbles will lead to a distorted image being obtained as a result of sound waves being blocked. A 60-ml syringe is attached to the small tap at the junction of the handle and shaft, which is filled with either degassed water or glycine. The transducer head can be filled in two ways:

1. By screwing the hard cone in place and slowly introducing the fluid from the syringe into the cone;
2. Opening the tap valve and flushing fluid through the shaft, then closing the tap.

Immerse the cone in a reservoir of the fluid, then slide the transducer into the cone and screw in place.

If there are any air bubbles in the cone, they may be expelled by holding the probe in an upright position, and then pushing fluid through it via the syringe. The air escapes via a pinhole at the tip of the cone.

It is common practice to fit a condom over the cone and shaft to protect the instrument and reduce the needs for sterilization/ disinfection (Figure 8.3).

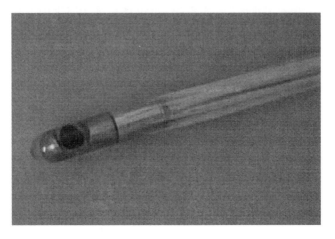

Figure 8.3 Hard plastic cone with outer protective condom.

After the procedure, the shaft and cone are wiped clean with an alcohol wipe or similar cleaning method, when a condom has been used to cover the probe. The probe should be taken apart at the end of the ultrasonography session, and the cone and shaft immersed in sterilizing fluid, following hospital guidelines. If a condom is not used during scanning, the probe should be disinfected and then sterilized after each use.

Method

The patient is normally in the left lateral position for the investigation. The probe is inserted up to approximately 4-5 cm from the anal verge, which can be determined by the graduations on the shaft. To yield images with a standard orientation, such that the top of the image obtained is anterior, the syringe needs to be upright while the patient is in the left lateral position. The probe is then slowly withdrawn into the anal canal, and the landmark of puborectalis identified. At this point the transducer is withdrawn further until the sling-type appearance changes into the external anal sphincter, which denotes the upper anal canal. An image is taken and stored onto disk, or as hard copy on print paper. The probe is withdrawn further until definition of the sphincters is lost (very close to or at the anal verge), and then slowly re-inserted until complete definition of the sphincters has been achieved; an image is taken at this point – low anal canal. The probe is then inserted further to obtain a midanal canal image. It is often necessary to pass the probe in and out of the anal canal several times throughout the examination, especially when assessing fistulae and abscesses.

On occasion it may not be possible to obtain a clear image of the sphincter complex with the patient in a resting state. Image enhancement may be achieved by asking the patient to perform a voluntary contraction (squeeze) of the anal sphincters. This will *sometimes* generate a more defined image of the sphincters[1, 2].

Ultrasonogram anatomy

Six ultrasonographic layers of the anal canal are visible when performing endoanal ultrasonography (Figure 8.4):

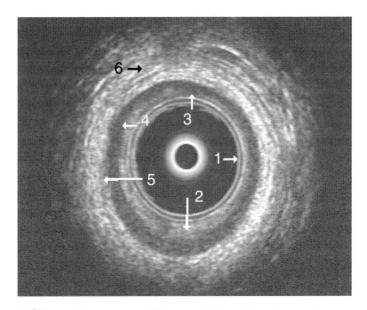

Figure 8.4 Normal ultrasonographic image of the anal canal musculature.

1. Interface of the cone and/or latex balloon: hyperechoic
2. Mucosa: hypoechoic
3. Subepithelial tissues: hyperechoic
4. Internal anal sphincter: hypoechoic
5. Intersphincteric plane and longitudinal muscle: hyperechoic
6. External anal sphincter (striated muscle): mixed echogenicity.

At the level of the upper anal canal, the external anal sphincter merges with puborectalis, which appears as a U shape and is hyperechoic. The vagina may also be visualized at this level. The anatomy and integrity of the anal sphincter complex are probably best visualized in the midanal canal, because the upper anal canal is most often misinterpreted by the untrained person.[3]

The intersphincteric plane is most clearly seen at the low anal canal level, which contains the subcutaneous fragment of the external anal sphincter. It is essential when performing endoanal ultrasonography that each of these three levels is clearly visualized in order to obtain a clear view of the anatomy, with all images clearly labelled. It is also possible to video the ultrasonographic study and review it at a later stage with the referring consultant.

When assessing anal fistulae, it is possible to highlight the tract by injection of hydrogen peroxide into the external opening, or by positioning a blunt-tipped needle within the sinus. Various studies have been performed with regard to this procedure.[4] The fistulous tract will then appear as a bright or hyperechoic streak during anal ELUS imaging. Without enhancement of the tract, it will be seen as a hypoechoic tract. It is important to identify the presence or absence of an internal opening into the anal canal through the sphincters and mucosa if possible.

The boundaries of the anal sphincter in women may also be defined by inserting the index finger into the vagina and pressing on the posterior vaginal wall. The finger is then highlighted as a hyperechoic U-shaped ridge, which outlines the posterior vaginal wall. This can be difficult to perform because of entrapment of air within the vagina, which yields a poor image.

Normal endoanal ultrasonography

When cylindrical longitudinal images of endoanal scans created by three-dimensional representation software package were studied in nulliparous and normal female volunteers, a natural gap was found in the external anal sphincter (EAS) below the level of puborectalis in all volunteers and 75 per cent of nulliparous women; manometry provided confirmation of the gaps seen[5] (Figure 8.5). The female sphincter, therefore, has a variable natural defect occurring along the anterior length, which makes interpretation of the isolated endoluminal ultrasonography difficult and may explain previous over-reporting of obstetric sphincter defects.

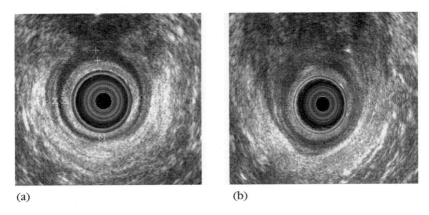

(a) (b)

Figure 8.5 (a) Anatomical defect; (b) external anal sphincter traumatic defect. Characteristic differences between anatomical defects and sphincter trauma: Normal, anteriorly; uniform hypoechogenicity, edges smooth and uniform, symmetrical. Ruptured sphincter/trauma, anteriorly; mixed echogenicity, edges ragged and irregular, asymmetrical.

When measured in asymptomatic individuals, the internal anal sphincter (IAS) thickness shows no difference with regard to gender; the EAS, however, has in a few studies been shown to be thicker in men than in women[6], although most studies show no difference. The EAS becomes thinner with age, unlike the IAS, which appears to become thicker with age. EAS thickness has been found to correlate inversely with IAS thickness.

Childbirth and the anal canal

The passage of the fetal head through the pelvis during childbirth obviously causes marked stretching of the tissues around the vagina and anal canal. Tissue and nerve damage is caused by either direct pressure or over-stretching and, in time, secondary muscle wasting occurs as a result of denervation. Although we have been able to study the effects of nerve damage on the anal sphincter for some time, it is only with the advent of endoanal sonography that we have been able to visualize the sphincter itself and the changes that occur in it during childbirth.

We have no good evidence that pregnancy itself changes the appearance or function of the anal sphincter. Rather it is during the process of labour and delivery itself that damage may occur. This is supported by the fact that women delivered by elective caesarean section report no change in their bowel habit[7]. However, it has been shown that 35 per cent of women delivering vaginally for the first time developed anal sphincter defects and that 13 per cent of the same group had problems with the control of their bowel[8]. The same study showed that 44 per cent of multigravidae had sphincter defects and 23 per cent were symptomatic. When women have been followed through two vaginal deliveries, it was found that, although the risk of sphincter injury is greatest after the first childbirth, a second delivery was found to place the women at high risk of worsening any bowel symptoms already present[9].

If we accept that problems of bowel control after vaginal delivery are much more common than previously estimated, greater efforts have to be made to detect women who are at risk. There is still a taboo over problems of faecal incontinence[10]. Although women are now increasingly willing to consult their general practitioner about urinary incontinence, they are much less likely to volunteer information about faecal symptoms. Indeed they will often deny any such difficulties, even on direct questioning. Clearly there is a need for the implementation of an improvement in public education.

However, as professionals we have to make much greater efforts to raise the issue with patients, to question them directly on bowel problems, and to institute the necessary investigations and follow-up when needed. Health workers have to be better informed of these issues and a system for referral, investigation and treatment should be in place for women with bowel symptoms or recognized sphincter damage.

Midwives and doctors should be trained in the detection of anal sphincter tears at the time of delivery. A rectal examination should be done if there is any suggestion of sphincter damage. Ideally, endoanal ultrasonography should be done as soon after delivery as possible. Obviously this facility will not be available in every unit and the patient may need to be referred to a specialist centre. Endoanal ultrasonography has been shown to be more sensitive than anorectal physiology in the detection of sphincter defects[11], and is therefore the initial investigation of choice. At the very least, however, women with sphincter damage should be reviewed at the hospital postnatally, and questioned about their bowel habits, something that until recently many units have been very poor at.

The incidence of bowel problems after delivery is grossly underestimated because affected women are reluctant to present to their doctors. Endoluminal ultrasonography, by detecting sphincter damage, allows us to monitor those patients at risk of developing problems of bowel control. We should remember that not all women with defects on the EAS will have problems immediately. They may develop symptoms over the years, with progressive atrophy of their tissues, perhaps compounded by a reduction in the function of the nerve supply to the pelvic muscles, causing them to suffer incontinence at a later date.

Relationship with anal manometry and neurophysiological assessments[12]

The sum of the thickness of the sphincters has been found to correlate with resting pressures, thus reflecting their tonic activity. Other studies found an inverse correlation between the sonographic thickness of the IAS and the resting anal tone in patients with intact sphincters. As clinical diagnosis can be difficult in differentiating between traumatic and idiopathic faecal incontinence, ELUS provides additional information about the sphincters, whilst pudendal nerve terminal motor latency (PNTML) can reveal unsuspected neuropathy in traumatic incontinence; thus, the combination of ELUS and PNTML is useful in selecting patients for surgery.

Anorectal disease and endoanal ultrasonography[13]

Endoanal ultrasonography has been used in the evaluation of a wide variety of anorectal disorders.

Incontinence

Endoluminal ultrasonography is most widely used in the assessment of faecal incontinence. It reliably identifies both external and internal anal sphincters. Lesions of the EAS are defined as a disturbance of the normal hyperechoic ring (layer 6) outside the hypoechoic IAS. Lesions of the IAS, similarly, are seen as a disturbance of the normal hypoechoic ring (layer 4). It is 90–95 per cent accurate in detecting anal sphincter defects[14, 15]. In a study of 44 patients, the findings at ELUS were compared with those at operation; all 23 EAS defects were demonstrated[16]. Any 'thinning' of the sphincters can also be accurately seen and measured.

Assessment of complex sphincteric defects in patients with faecal incontinence by digital rectal examination and intraoperative dissection can be difficult in the presence of excessive scarring. Adjunctive investigations are useful. Endoluminal ultrasonography has replaced electromyographic sphincter mapping, which, though accurate, is a painful and time-consuming procedure[17]. Endovaginal endosonography has not been found to be helpful or accurate for assessing anal sphincter defects, because the distance between the transducer and the sphincter is increased, and the device is angulated to the axis of the anal canal. The value of transperineal sonography is not established because of lack of adequate data[18].

Endoluminal ultrasonography has brought new insight into the pathophysiological mechanisms of incontinence. It is helpful in the selection of patients with traumatic incontinence for sphincter repair. Unsuspected sphincter damage has been noted in a significant number of patients considered to have idiopathic incontinence. In neurogenic faecal incontinence, there is denervation of the EAS and pelvic floor muscles. This is often associated with changes in the IAS, which can be seen on ELUS[19]. Also, the ratio of the thickness of the EAS and IAS muscles may be reduced in patients with neurogenic incontinence compared with controls[20].

In the absence of denervation, structural damage, EAS weakness or sensory abnormalities, faecal incontinence may be associated with a thin hypoechogenic IAS with a poorly defined edge; the normal increase in IAS thickness with age is not seen. This primary degeneration of the IAS smooth muscle is a discrete clinical condition causing passive faecal incontinence[21]. The volume of the EAS–IAS complex (measured using three-dimensional ELUS) has been used as a parameter for continence outcome in childhood.

Constipation

The role of endoanal ultrasonography in constipation has been investigated. Both internal and external sphincter hypertrophy may be seen in some patients with obstructed defecation. Occasionally, IAS myopathy may be identified in patients with intractable constipation or proctalgia. In solitary rectal ulcer syndrome, sphincter hypertrophy may be seen.

Perianal sepsis and fistulae

In perianal sepsis, endoanal ultrasonography can reveal the site and presence of abscesses and fistulae, identifying the inner opening and the involvement of sphincter structures. This is useful in planning the most appropriate treatment – medical or surgical. The definition of fistula tract anatomy greatly assists accurate preoperative assessment. Visualization of complicated and recurrent fistula tracts can be achieved with the use of contrast agents as well as hydrogen peroxide[4]. Endoanal ultrasonography can diagnose, localize and define any extensions of perirectal abscesses[22]; it is an important therapeutic tool as well in aiding echo-guided drainage.

Congenital anorectal anomalies

Endoanal ultrasonography also plays an important role in the evaluation of patients with congenital anorectal anomalies, particularly in identifying the sphincteric mechanism before and after surgery for imperforate anus and cloacal defects. In rectovaginal fistulae, endoanal ultrasonography is recommended preoperatively to identify and map occult sphincter defects. This would aid concomitant anal sphincter reconstruction in patients with an endoanal ultrasonographically documented sphincter defect[23].

Trauma

Obstetric trauma is discussed separately. Endoanal ultrasonography is useful in evaluating and following up patients with sphincter injury secondary to blunt trauma. It has been found helpful in the evaluation of patients with anorectal complaints after haemorrhoidectomy and bowel surgery[24].

Miscellaneous

Endoanal ultrasonography can be used to follow up the anal sphincters of patients who have undergone 'dynamic stimulated gracilis neosphincter' surgery, providing an accurate assessment of the relationship between the neosphincter and the residual sphincter complex[25].

Anal carcinoma

Besides digital examination and proctoscopy with biopsy, endoanal ultrasonography complements the diagnosis of primary anal carcinoma[26]. The depth of infiltration can be determined in relation to the normal layers of the anal canal; in addition, enlarged lymph nodes in the pelvis may be visualized using endoanal ultrasonography. This allows accurate preoperative staging of squamous cell carcinoma of the anal canal. Follow-up after treatment is also possible.

Endorectal ultrasonography

The technique of endorectal ultrasonography differs from that of endoanal ultrasonography. The set-up of the transducer head requires a latex balloon to be fitted securely over the transducer with two connecting rings. This balloon is filled with between 40 and 60 ml of degassed water or glycine. The balloon is initially filled before insertion and then deflated in order to remove any air bubbles that may be present. Preferably a condom should also be placed over the probe and secured.

The patient can be prepared using a disposable enema, which can be patient administered, or a glycerin suppository – the guidelines that are in place for performing flexible sigmoidoscopy will be sufficient. The probe is introduced into the rectum with the patient in either the left lateral or the lithotomy position if performed in theatre for assessment of painful lesions, etc. The probe is guided to a position above the lesion if possible. The balloon is then inflated and the scanning commenced. It is often more practical to increase the image scale to yield a clearer image that includes the rectal wall and surrounding tissues. Images are taken throughout the rectum and labelled according to the height from the anal verge. The area of the lesion is assessed and images are obtained which will identify position and invasion of the tumour. It is often better to obtain videotapes of endorectal scans that identify lesions. It is not always possible to scan above 15 cm and, where resistance and/or pain is identified by the patient, the procedure may be performed under an anaesthetic.

In some instances it may be easier to perform the procedure with the use of a sigmoidoscope, which is inserted initially with the transducer being passed within. This enables the procedure to be done under full view.

Rectal wall anatomy

Upon endosonography, the rectal wall should have five distinguishable layers, of which two are hypoechoic and three hyperechoic (Figure 8.6). The visualization of the layers as described in this figure is essential in the staging of rectal lesions. The volume of water used within the balloon is adjusted accordingly during scanning to obtain the clearest image. This volume may be up to 120 ml.

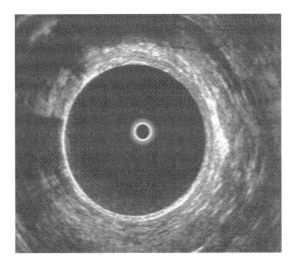

Figure 8.6 The five layers of the rectal wall, distinguishable by endosonography. The large black circle at the centre of the image is the water-filled balloon. The primary layer (hyperechoic) is the interface of the water, balloon and mucosa of the rectal wall. Adjacent to this layer is the mucosa (hypoechoic), followed by the interface of the mucosa, submucosa and muscularis propria (hyperechoic). The following hypoechoic layer represents the muscularis propria, which is adjacent to the interface between muscularis and fat (hyperechoic).

The anatomy within the pelvis can be identified during the investigation. The pelvic floor muscles (levator ani and coccygeus) are visible when the probe is positioned in the upper anal canal. The male bladder can be visualized, but its appearance is dependent on the fluid retained in it. The prostate is also visible – with a clear kidney-shaped outline – being hypoechoic in appearance. Bright spots (echoes) may be visible, which represent calcification. At a position just below the prostate, it is sometimes possible to visualize the urethra. In women the vagina is seen anteriorly to the rectum as a hypoechoic ellipse with hyperechoic wall.

With the balloon fully expanded, it may be necessary to change the frequency of the ultrasonic scanner. The rectal wall may be outwith the focal length of the 10 MHz scanner and a 7 or 5 MHz scanner may be required, although there is a loss of definition in the layers of the rectal wall when these changes have to be made.

In addition, for staging a rectal tumour, it is also useful and possible to attempt lymph node staging. For this the frequency of the ultrasonic scanner will definitely have to be stepped down to visualize out to the lateral pelvic side wall. It is noted that the involvement of any visualized lymph nodes is notoriously difficult to predict, not only using ultrasonography but also using computed tomography (CT) and magnetic resonance imaging (MRI). For the moment the most useful indicator of involved lymph nodes is a size greater than 5 mm.

Staging of rectal cancers

Rectal and colon cancers are usually staged using Dukes' classification, but it is more appropriate in this day and age to use the international TNM staging. M staging is not possible using the endorectal scanner because this indicates metastatic disease. T staging relates to the depth of tumour invasion of the bowel wall: T1 cancers are limited to the bowel mucosa; T2 disease breaches the muscularis propria of the bowel wall; T3 disease invades completely through the muscularis propria; and T4 disease involves adjacent organs. N staging is quite complex when reported by the pathologist or by the radiologist using MRI or CT. A differential is made between the involvement of local nodes and distant nodes. The lymph node pathways of the rectum mean that drainage is generally up the inferior mesenteric artery to the aorta, and this is well out of the range of endorectal ultrasonography. It is usual that only local nodes can be seen and therefore any positive nodes, usually by the size test, are reported simply as N1.

The importance of this staging relates to treatment pathways. Disease restricted to the bowel wall with no evidence of lymph node invasion is often operated on as the primary mode of treatment, whereas disease that penetrates through the full thickness of the bowel wall (T3) and which may involve adjacent organs (T4), or disease in which there are positive lymph nodes, is often treated initially by chemoradiotherapy or radiotherapy alone to downstage a tumour and limit local recurrence.

Follow-up

Endorectal ultrasonography has two uses in follow-up. The first is in reassessment of tumour and nodal disease after treatment with primary radiotherapy; the scan is undertaken before surgery to view the degree of down-staging that has been achieved. The second is in following up patients who have had resection and anastomosis in an attempt to identify early tumour recurrence at the anastomotic line. If this modality of follow-up is used it is important to get the surgeon to document the level of anastomosis accurately, so that the appropriate area can be scanned.

Conclusion

The technique of endoanal ultrasonography is appealing for a number of reasons. It is a non-invasive procedure and does not involve the patient being subjected to any radiation. The technique can usually be adequately performed within the laboratory or examination room setting, but may also be used in conjunction with surgical procedures in the operating theatre. Although the initial outlay for the system is not inexpensive, the scope and worth of the procedure make it economical. The procedure itself is generally well tolerated in most patients, other than the patients previously highlighted, yielding less discomfort than a routine digital examination. The technique is relatively simple to learn and put into practice.

The use of ELUS in the anal region is primarily to evaluate patients with incontinence, either traumatic or idiopathic. It has gained an important position as a diagnostic test in the evaluation of the anatomical condition of the anal sphincters. It is less painful than and superior to electromyography in identifying defects in the EAS. Endosonography may complement nerve conduction studies, and it has been proposed to be the only other test needed besides physical examination to evaluate the status of the IAS.

Its ultimate role in the evaluation of certain anal conditions is likely to improve with advances in ultrasonographic technology, which are on the horizon. This will especially hold true as clinicians and ultrasonographers become more familiar with the performance of ELUS studies.

Instrument design limits endoanal ultrasonography to the axial plane; however, three-dimensional reconstructions have been used to explore sex differences in anal canal and sphincter length, as well as the relationship between the radial and linear extent of any anal sphincter tear.[27]

Recently, endoanal MRI has been compared with endoanal ultrasonography and appears to provide accurate information on the extent and structure of complex sphincter lesions.[28] The practicality of this application may, however, be hindered by the increasing demands being put on MRI, and hence it may be difficult to negotiate sufficient time for anal sphincter observation. The waiting time for endoanal ultrasonography is likely to be significantly less, as is the actual procedure time. However, there are certain instances that may require MRI in addition to standard endoanal ultrasonography.

References

1. Rieger NA, Downey PR, Wattchow DA. Endo-anal ultrasound during contraction of the anal sphincter - improved definition and diagnostic accuracy. Br J Radiol 1996; 69: 665–667
2. Frudinger A, Bartram CI, Halligan S, Kamm MA. Examination techniques for endosonography of the anal canal. Abdom imaging 1998; 23: 301–303
3. Enck P, Heyer T, Gantle B et al. How reproducible are measures of the anal sphincter muscle diameter by endoanal ultrasound? Dis Colon Rectum 1998; 41: 1000–1004
4. Cheong DM, Nogueras JJ, Wexner SD, Jagelman DG. Anal endosonography for recurrent anal fistulas: image enhancement with hydrogen peroxide. Dis Colon Rectum 1993; 36: 1158–1160
5. Bollard RC, Gardiner A, Lindow S, Phillips K, Duthie GS. Normal women have natural anal sphincter defects. Dis Colon Rectum 2003; in press
6. Papachrysostomou M, Pye SD, Smith AN. Anal endosonography in asymptomatic subjects. Scand J Gastroenterol 1993; 28: 551–556
7. Fynes M, Donnelly VS, O'Connell PR, O'Herlihy C. Caesarean delivery and anal sphincter injury. Obstet Gynaecol 1998; 92 (4 Pt 1): 496–500
8. Sultan AH, Kamm MA, Hudson CN, Thomas JM, Bartram CI. Anal sphincter disruption during vaginal delivery. N Engl J Med 1993; 329: 1905–1911
9. Fynes M, Donnelly V, Behan M, O'Connell PR, O'Herlihy C. Effect of second vaginal delivery on anorectal physiology and faecal incontinence: a prospective study. Lancet 1999; 354: 965–966
10. Burnett SJD, Spence-Jones C, Speakman CTM, Kamm MA, Hudson CN, Bartram CI. Unsuspected sphincter damage following childbirth revealed by anal endosonography. Br J Radiol 1991; 64: 225–227
11. Favetta U, Amato A, Interisano A, Pescatori M. Clinical, manometric and sonographic assessment of the anal sphincters. A comparative prospective study. Int J Colorectal Dis 1996; 11: 163–166

12. Felt-Bersma RJ, Cuesta MA, Koorevaar M, Strijers RL, Meuwissen SG, Dercksen EJ. Anal endosonography: relationship with anal manometry and neurophysiologic tests. Dis Colon Rectum 1992; 35: 944-949

13. Poen AC, Felt-Bersma RJ. Endosonography in benign anorectal disease: an overview. Scand J Gastroenterol Suppl 1999; 230: 40-48

14. Law PJ, Kamm MA, Bartram CI. Anal endosonography in the investigation of faecal incontinence. Br J Surg 1991; 78: 312-314

15. Cuesta MA, Meijer S, Derksen EJ, Boutkan H, Meuwissen SG. Anal sphincter imaging in faecal incontinence using endosonography. Dis Colon Rectum 1992; 35: 59-63

16. Meyenberger C, Bertschinger P, Zala GF, Buchmann P. Anal sphincter defects in faecal incontinence: correlation between endosonography and surgery. Endoscopy 1996; 28: 217-224

17. Tjandra JJ, Milsom JW, Fazio VW. Endoluminal ultrasound is preferable to electromyography in mapping anal sphincter defects. Dis Col Rectum 1993; 36: 689-692

18. Rubens DJ, Strang JG, Bogineni-Misra S, Wexler IE. Transperineal sonography of the rectum: anatomy and pathology revealed by sonography compared with CT and MR imaging. Am J Gastroenterol 1998; 170: 637-642

19. Lubowski DZ, Nicholls RJ, Burleigh DE, Swash M. Internal anal sphincter in neurogenic faecal incontinence. Gastroenterology 1988; 95: 997-1002

20. Emblem R, Dhaenens G, Stien R, Morkrid L, Aasen AO, Bergan R. The importance of anal endosonography in the evaluation of idiopathic faecal incontinence. Dis Colon Rectum 1994; 37: 42-48

21. Vaizey CJ, Kamm MA, Bartram CI. Primary degeneration of the internal anal sphincter as a cause of passive faecal incontinence. Lancet 1997; 349: 612-615

22. Lobo Martinez E, Torres Aleman A, Galindo Alvarez J, Martinez Molina E. Endoanal ultrasound in perirectal abscesses. Rev Esp Enferm Dig 1997; 89: 897-902

23. Yee LF, Birnbaum EH, Read TE, Kodner IJ, Fleshman JW. Use of endoanal ultrasound in patients with rectovaginal fistulas. Dis Colon Rectum 1999; 42: 1057-1064

24. Farouk R, Duthie GS, Lee PW, Monson JR. Endosonographic evidence of injury to the internal anal sphincter after low anterior resection: long term follow-up. Dis Colon Rectum 1998; 41: 888-891

25. Marano I, Grassi R, Donnianni T et al. CT and anal endosonography in the evaluation of electrically stimulated neosphincter: a preliminary report. Abdom Imaging 1996; 21: 353-356

26. Herzog U, Boss M, Spichtin HP. Endoanal ultrasonography in the follow-up of anal carcinoma. Surg Endosc 1994; 8: 1186-1189

27. Gold DM, Bartram CI, Halligan S, Humphries KN, Kamm MA, Kmiot WA. Three dimensional endoanal sonography in assessing anal canal injury. Br J Surg 1999; 86: 365-370

28. Rociu E, Stoker J, Eijkemans MJ, Schouten WR, Lameris JS. Faecal incontinence: endoanal US versus endoanal MR imaging. Radiology 1999; 212: 453-458

Chapter 9
Biofeedback and anorectal disease

AMANDA ROY

Biofeedback

The theoretical basis for biofeedback is learning through reinforcement. It is a re-education tool whereby information about a specific physiological function is relayed to a patient in real time so that the patient can act upon the information to make positive changes. Biofeedback was first applied in clinical psychology for teaching muscle relaxation and stress management, but has since been used for modification of autonomic functions such as blood pressure in hypertension, pulmonary function in people with asthma, vascular function in migraine headache and motor function in neuromuscular rehabilitation.

Increasingly, over the past 20 years, biofeedback techniques have also been used to treat patients with defecatory disorders. Initially incontinence, then constipation and more recently irritable bowel syndrome (IBS) have been treated with biofeedback. Biofeedback techniques can be applied to defecation because there are conscious, modifiable elements involved in the defecatory process, such as anal sphincter contraction and relaxation, propulsive effort and awareness of rectal contents. Although biofeedback may focus on a specific physical aspect of defecation, such as strengthening or relaxing certain muscles, it would be a gross over-simplification to try to correlate any one physiological measurement to a psychofunctional process such as defecation. For this reason, both subjective and objective assessments have often been found to correlate poorly with physiological measurements before and after biofeedback; as a consequence the mechanisms by which biofeedback works have been difficult to define.

Incontinence

The most commonly reported use of biofeedback techniques is in the treatment of faecal incontinence[1]. Faecal incontinence is defined as 'the involuntary or inappropriate passage of faeces'[2]. It is a disruptive condition that can disable patients socially and psychologically. The cause of faecal incontinence in women relates primarily to traumatic vaginal delivery, with 4 per cent of women experiencing at least one episode of frank faecal incontinence after their first vaginal delivery[3]. There are, however, many medical and surgical causes of incontinence in both men and women, and faecal incontinence affects over 1 per cent of the adult population[4]. Faecal incontinence can arise as a result of damaged anal sphincters or may occur in the presence of a normal sphincter if the stool is liquid or the bowel contracts vigorously[5].

In the past, treatment options for faecal incontinence have been limited to either surgery or constipating drugs. For those with frank incontinence and discrete external anal sphincter defects that can be localized on endoanal ultrasonography, surgical repair is usually indicated[1]. Anterior sphincter repair may help most patients in the short term[6]. Post-anal repair, which attempts to restore the anorectal angle by plication of the pelvic floor muscles behind the sphincter, has been shown to improve the degree of continence in less than 50 per cent of patients[7], and efficacy has been shown to be poor in the long term[8]. More radical and invasive surgical options include the formation of a neosphincter, most commonly using the gracilis muscle, the use of an artificial sphincter or the formation of a stoma. Where there is internal anal sphincter damage for which there is no effective surgical procedure, sphincter weakness but no apparent structural damage, or for those with urgency but a normal sphincter, the use of a constipating agent such as loperamide may control passive seepage by making the stool firmer. There is also some evidence that loperamide directly reduces the sensation of urgency[9] and increases resting anal sphincter tone. Biofeedback techniques alone may be undertaken as a first-line treatment or in addition to these other treatment options. Even in patients with a surgically repairable lesion, residual functional capacity may be improved with biofeedback therapy to bring about symptomatic improvement[10]. Although it is still unclear how it works and evaluation is difficult as a result of the different techniques and outcome measures used, published studies show an improvement in 50–92 per cent of patients[11].

The number and length of each biofeedback session differ from centre to centre, but generally begin with an assessment interview so that patients are able to discuss their symptoms in detail. As a result of the embarrassing nature of faecal incontinence, many individuals may never have fully discussed their condition. Information on normal bowel control and the maintenance of continence may be provided using pictures or anatomical models, and the results of any previous investigations such as endoanal ultrasonography or sphincter manometry may be explained.

One of the main elements of biofeedback for faecal incontinence is teaching patients how to isolate, coordinate and strengthen the anal sphincters. Kegel first described the effects of pelvic floor exercises on stress urinary incontinence. Studies have since shown that biofeedback is superior to Kegel exercises alone in faecal incontinence.[11] The teaching method and the number and type of exercises differ considerably between studies. However, in general, sphincter exercises are demonstrated using computer-assisted visual (or sometimes audio-) feedback from electromyography (EMG) probes on the skin at each side of the anus, or from an EMG or manometry probe placed in the anal canal[10, 12]. The patient observes the changes in the trace on the computer screen when asked to squeeze his or her anal sphincter. Maximal, submaximal, rapid and prolonged squeezes may be undertaken, and often patients are provided with a set of sphincter exercises to complete at home. In other studies, patients have been given portable biofeedback equipment to use at home. Encouragement and motivation are vital because the patient may be asked to undertake numerous exercises several times a day.

Studies by Delechenaut et al.[13] and Engel et al.[14] have emphasized the relationship between sphincter pressures and incontinence. Patients with passive faecal incontinence have significantly lower anal sphincter resting pressures, and patients with urge incontinence are characterized by lower voluntary contraction pressures. However, the interrelationship of clinical symptoms, anorectal pathophysiology and the results of biofeedback has been poorly characterized. Most studies have reported that efficacy is not predictable based on anorectal resting or squeeze pressures before or after treatment[11]. Some authors have reported no change in resting or squeeze pressure with biofeedback[15, 16], whereas others have shown a strengthening effect[17, 18], and there have also been suggestions that sphincter symmetry may be important[19]. Glia et al.[20] showed that there was greater radial asymmetry of the anal sphincter in those patients not responding to biofeedback. There has also been interest in strengthening the anal sphincter using electrical stimulation, and Fynes et al.[21] reported an increased rate of success using conventional biofeedback techniques augmented with electrical stimulation of the anal sphincter.

Studies have shown that sensitivity to rectal distension may also determine continence and biofeedback outcome[22,23], and consequently rectal sensitivity training has been incorporated into biofeedback training to help the patient identify the presence of stool in the rectum and to coordinate contraction of the external sphincter with reflex relaxation of the internal sphincter. Maximum tolerated volume reflects rectal storage capacity, so trying to increase the maximum tolerated volume has been the focus for some studies. Rectal sensitivity training often consists of inserting a balloon into the rectum and gradually inflating the balloon until the patient reports the urge to defecate. Increasing amounts of air or water are introduced into the balloon for prolonged intervals and the patient is advised to contract their external sphincter in response to the urge to defecate. The patient learns to relax and to suppress the feeling of urgency. Gradually the patient becomes able to defer defecation for longer periods as a result of desensitization of the rectum and coordination of the anal sphincters. Conversely, for those with an insensitive rectum the aim is to increase sensitivity using progressively lower volumes of balloon distension in the rectum[10].

The maintenance of continence is a complex process depending not only on sphincter function but also on stool consistency, colonic and rectal function and psychological state; because of this a package of care needs to be provided that is tailored to the individual patient's needs. Thus evaluation of treatment is further complicated by the fact that a session of biofeedback may involve other elements, in addition to sphincter exercises and rectal sensitivity training. Additional measures consist of general education about normal bowel habit, counselling and support, dietary advice (including reduction of fibre and caffeine), personal cleaning and odour advice, and use of anti-diarrhoeals such as loperamide capsules or syrup to improve stool consistency. Despite problems with the comparison of studies, biofeedback has consistently been shown in published studies to be an effective treatment option for patients with faecal incontinence.

Constipation

Many patients with the subjective complaint of constipation are resistant to laxatives and experience major physical, social, and psychological impairment from their condition. The great majority of these patients in the UK are female[24]. The process of defecation involves learning to use the skeletal muscles of the pelvic floor and anal sphincter. Once children learn to contract these muscles to maintain continence they must also learn to inhibit contraction to allow defecation. Inappropriate pelvic floor contraction in many constipated patients during attempted defecation formed the original focus for biofeedback, and it has now become a well-established technique with more than half of all adult patients responding favourably[25].

Biofeedback for constipation was first described by Bleijenberg and Kuijpers, when it was performed over a protracted inpatient stay and associated with a success rate of 70 per cent[26]. Since this time, problems have arisen concerning the terminology used in this area. A variety of terms is used in the literature to describe evacuation disorders. These include anismus, pelvic floor dysfunction, paradoxical puborectalis contraction, puborectalis dyssynergia and spastic pelvic floor syndrome. The term 'obstructed defecation' is also used when a patient needs to strain or digitate to aid evacuation, although no physical obstruction is present. To complicate matters further, some findings that are reported as abnormal, such as failure to open the anorectal angle and paradoxical contraction of the pelvic floor muscles, have been found in asymptomatic controls[27, 28]. In addition to difficulties in defining the patients being treated, evaluation of the efficacy of biofeedback in constipated patients has been hindered by the small number of patients in many studies, and differences in the method of treatment, outcome measures and length of follow-up. Despite these factors, however, biofeedback has consistently been shown to be effective in 40–60 per cent of patients, and more recent studies have demonstrated similar success rates when studying larger patient groups and long-term efficacy[25, 29]. Although initially only patients with paradoxical pelvic floor contraction and normal transit times were referred for biofeedback because of its success, patients with many other causes of constipation are now treated with this therapy. Patients treated with biofeedback techniques include not only those with no pelvic floor dysfunction or with slow transit constipation, but also those with rectoceles, rectal prolapse, increased perineal descent, rectoanal intussusception and rectal pain.

Most patients are treated on an outpatient basis. Generally the patient will see the same biofeedback therapist throughout treatment in order to establish a good patient–therapist relationship, which is necessary for positive reinforcement. A careful history and symptom assessment allow the patient the opportunity to talk at length about the problems. It has been shown that there is a high incidence of anxiety and psychological problems in patients with constipation, and up to 50 per cent of patients presenting with idiopathic constipation may have a background of childhood bereavement or abuse[30]. Some authors feel that these issues should be addressed directly, and Leroi et al.[31] have shown that the combination of psychotherapy and biofeedback can be a useful approach. However, the biofeedback session can provide a sympathetic setting for discussing problems without addressing psychological problems directly. This can overcome the tendency observed by Drossman[32] for patients to see a suggestion that their problem is psychological as a rejection. The counselling offered in biofeedback may allow patients to come to this conclusion themselves in a neutral context.

Normal colonic function and the defecatory process can be explained to the patient with the aid of diagrams. Patients may be advised to sit comfortably on the toilet with their feet raised slightly and their arms resting on their thighs, and discouraged from adopting unusual positions on the toilet. Patients who do not have a helpful defecatory routine, perhaps because they dread defecation or spend an inordinately long time on the toilet straining without success, may be advised to adopt a more helpful daily routine. Treatment must be tailored to the patient so that those spending hours, several times a day, on the toilet are told to attempt defecation less frequently and those going once a week are advised to practise defecatory exercises daily. It may be useful to advise patients to attempt defecation at a set time each day in order to establish a routine, and they are often advised to choose a time shortly after eating so as to coincide with the gastrocolic reflex. In some studies advice about laxatives is given and decreasing laxative use may be used as an outcome measure. Alternatively patients may be advised to stop laxatives before the onset of therapy so that both the severity of the problem and any changes with treatment can be assessed. This may take a great effort on the part of the patient who may have taken a particular laxative as a routine over many years. It may be useful to advise patients that their problem, often a very long-standing one, will not be solved overnight but, with due use of the strategies taught, they will improve.

In addition to the education and advice given to patients, the number of sessions, length of the sessions and time between sessions differ considerably between studies. All modalities of treatment initially focus on teaching the patient to relax the pelvic floor during defecatory straining, but in most studies other variables are also associated with the treatment. Constipation is a psychofunctional abnormality and cannot be reduced to a simple manometric abnormality; most patients are able to learn how to relax their anal sphincter in the laboratory setting, whereas only some are cured of their symptoms[33]. A correlation has, however, been shown between a successful outcome with biofeedback and change in autonomic function. Using laser Doppler rectal mucosal blood flow, biofeedback was shown to modify central autonomic control of colonic function in constipated patients[34].

To teach appropriate pelvic floor relaxation most studies use sphincter EMG as the feedback signal because this can be conveniently performed with surface EMG electrodes, which are placed on the pelvic floor at each side of the anus. It is therefore a non-invasive and thus less threatening procedure for the patient. Often colourful traces and graphs are used to demonstrate sphincter activity but, as with biofeedback for incontinence, different teaching aids and different computer programs are used in different studies. The general concept is that, on squeezing the sphincter, patients observe an increase in activity, and on bearing down they should observe a decrease in activity brought about by the relaxation of the anal sphincter and pelvic floor, which is necessary for normal defecation. To aid this process many studies also simulate defecation by asking the patient to attempt to expel a rectal balloon. Ability to expel the balloon demonstrates not only pelvic floor relaxation but also whether there is sufficient propulsive force for defecation, coordinated with the sphincter relaxation. Expulsion of a balloon may also enable patients to see that they are making progress, especially if symptoms persist. Patients may be taught to avoid tensing up at the thought of having to defecate, via relaxation breathing. Patients therefore learn to evacuate stool as easily and effectively as possible by remaining relaxed, pushing effectively, and relaxing rather than contracting the anal sphincter.

Patients may be given specific instructions and defecatory exercises which must be practised at home; in some centres a portable biofeedback unit is given to the patient for use at home. The session can be tailored to the particular patient, with more emphasis on pelvic floor relaxation in patients with inappropriate sphincter contraction, and more emphasis on behavioural modification in those with unusual or unhelpful toileting habits.

Normal toileting is not simply a matter of learning to respond to bladder or bowel pressures by relaxing the pelvic floor, but is a complex operant and social learning process[35]. Thus, as with biofeedback for incontinence, biofeedback therapy for constipation involves other elements, and several studies have emphasized that there are many aspects to treatment other than the biofeedback technique itself[25,29]. As previously described, these may include symptomatic assessment, counselling, health education, coordination exercises, behavioural therapy and the use of relaxation techniques.

For constipation, biofeedback is the only option other than continued laxative use or continued symptoms. Only a small minority of patients will be suitable for surgical intervention (usually colectomy and ileorectal anastomosis). Resolution of specific symptoms, such as abdominal pain and bloating, is unpredictable and there is a risk of postoperative complications such as diarrhoea and impaired continence[36]. Bernini et al.[37] evaluated patients with intractable constipation who had undergone subtotal colectomy between 1982 and 1995, and reported that almost half were dissatisfied with their surgery. Surgery should be considered only in patients with severe complaints and after extensive physiological and psychological evaluation[38]. Past surgical treatments for obstructed defecation have included division of the puborectalis muscle[39] and anorectal myectomy[40], but these treatments are not effective and carry a risk of incontinence. Other options may include psychotherapy, hypnotherapy and non-specific relaxation techniques such as yoga. Guthrie et al.[41] found that psychotherapy improved symptoms of IBS except for constipation and Wise et al.[42] reported that group therapy reduced constipation in only 15 per cent of patients with severe symptoms despite marked improvement in psychometric scores. Likewise, yoga has been shown to be less effective than biofeedback[43].

Despite its reported success, the mode of action of biofeedback therapy in constipated patients is still unclear. A study looking at the results of biofeedback therapy in 194 patients with constipation treated over a 9-year period attempted not only to determine efficacy, but also to try to identify predictors of success[29]. Age, gender, duration of symptoms, degree of perineal descent, presence or absence of rectocele, presence or absence of rectoanal intussusception, mean or maximum resting or squeeze pressure, sensory threshold and maximum tolerated volume all failed to predict outcome from therapy. The only predictor of success was found to be the patient's willingness to complete the course of treatment. Similar results were found for 100 patients in a study carried out at St Mark's Hospital, Northwick Park, Harrow[25]; biofeedback therapy was equally successful in slow and normal transit patients and those with and without paradoxical pelvic floor contraction, and anorectal physiology tests failed to predict outcome. In contrast Karlbom et al.[44] found that the severity of constipation and laxative use were possible predictors of outcome and McKee et al.,[24] following assessment of all patients by an evacuating proctogram, whole-gut transit and anorectal physiology, found that patients with abnormal pelvic floor physiology were less likely to benefit from biofeedback.

Abnormalities in distal colonic motility have also been reported in a subset of patients with disordered evacuation[45]. This may represent a rectocolonic inhibitory reflex and could explain success with biofeedback. Stimulation of the rectum by retained stool or gas within the functionally obstructed rectum causes a reflex inhibition of the colon. Thus, restoration of normal evacuation using biofeedback would result in normalization of colonic motility.

Many factors may therefore be involved in the success or failure of biofeedback, including retraining and alteration of the mechanisms of defecation, behavioural changes and improved subjective well-being via the counselling and support of the patient–therapist relationship. Biofeedback for constipation has no side effects, is non-invasive and is relatively inexpensive, although it does require the significant time and expense of a dedicated therapist. It is successful in most patients and can be used as a first-line treatment for constipation.

Other indications

Biofeedback techniques may also have a role to play in the treatment of patients with IBS, although it has been used less frequently in this area. Again, treatment protocols vary. As with its use in constipation and incontinence, treatment may be centred on effective control of defecatory muscles and in overcoming blocks on proper bowel function that are related to the patient's lifestyle or psychological issues. In addition, biofeedback for IBS may focus more on relaxation. In one study[46], a computer biofeedback game was developed based on animated gut imagery in order to teach relaxation to IBS patients. Half the patients with refractory IBS found the treatment helpful.

Patients with solitary rectal ulcer syndrome have been treated with biofeedback alone, or in a combined approach with biofeedback undertaken before or immediately after surgery. Solitary rectal ulcer syndrome is uncommon and difficult to treat, and biofeedback retraining has been found to be a useful treatment in this condition[47].

Biofeedback techniques have also been found to be successful in specific patient groups with bowel problems, e.g. in children[48], elderly people[49] and individuals with learning difficulties[50]. Until the 1960s, it was assumed that people with severe learning disabilities could not be toilet trained. Continence makes a major difference to the life of the individual and the carers, and was shown to be the major consideration in deciding on the independence of the individual. It has been shown that behaviour modification methods, using positive reinforcement and biofeedback techniques, can be successfully used to teach toileting even to people with profound disabilities[50].

Conclusion

Despite many studies, the definitive mode of action of biofeedback therapy remains obscure, although it may include improvement in both motor and sensory functions of the anorectum in addition to behavioural modification via positive reinforcement and the support of the therapist. The universal features of biofeedback are that it is a morbidity-free, relatively non-invasive, well-tolerated, inexpensive outpatient treatment. Biofeedback techniques are now widely recognized as the treatment of choice in defecatory disorders.

References

1. Norton C. Faecal incontinence in adults 2: treatment and management. Br J Nursing 1997; 6: 23–26
2. Royal College of Physicians. Incontinence: Causes, Management and Provision of Services. London: Royal College of Physicians, 1995

3. Konsten J, Baeten CG, Havenith MG, Soeters PB. Morphology of dynamic graciloplasty compared with the anal sphincter. Dis Colon Rectum 1993; 36: 559-563

4. Nelson R, Norton N, Cautley E, Furner S. Community based prevalence of anal incontinence. JAMA 1995; 274: 559-561

5. Herbst F, Kamm MA, Morris GP, Britton K, Wolszko J, Nicholls RJ. Gastrointestinal transit and prolonged ambulatory colonic motility in health and faecal incontinence. Gut 1997; 41: 381-389

6. Engel AE, Kamm MA, Sultan AH, Bartram CI, Nicholls J. Anterior anal sphincter repair in patients with obstetric trauma. Br J Surg 1994; 81: 131-134

7. Van Tets WF, Kuijpers JHC. Pelvic floor procedures produce no consistent changes in anatomy or physiology. Dis Colon Rectum 1998; 41: 365-368

8. Jameson JS, Speakman CT, Darzi A, Chia YW, Henry MM. Audit of postanal repair in the treatment of faecal incontinence. Dis Colon Rectum 1994; 37: 33-72

9. Goke M, Ewe K, Donner K, Meyer zum Buschenfelde KH. Influence of loperamide and loperamide oxide on the anal sphincter; a manometric study. Dis Colon Rectum 1992; 35: 857-861

10. Norton C, Kamm MA. Outcome of biofeedback for faecal incontinence. Br J Surg 1999; 86: 1159-1163

11. Enck P. Biofeedback training in disordered defaecation: a critical review. Dig Dis Sci 1993; 38: 1953-1960

12. Fleshman JW, Dreznik Z, Meyer K et al. Outpatient protocol for biofeedback therapy of pelvic floor outlet obstruction. Dis Colon Rectum 1992; 35: 1-7

13. Delechenaut P, Leroi AM, Weber J, Touchais JY, Czernichow P, Denis P. Relationship between clinical symptoms of anal incontinence and the results of anorectal manometry. Dis Colon Rectum 1992; 35: 847-849

14. Engel AF, Kamm MA, Bartram CI, Nicholls RJ. Relationship of symptoms in faecal incontinence to specific sphincter abnormalities. Int J Colorectal Dis 1995; 30: 152-155

15. Loening-Baucke V. Efficacy of biofeedback training in improving faecal incontinence and anorectal physiology function. Gut 1990; 31: 1395-1402

16. Latimar PR, Campbell D, Kaperski J. A components analysis of biofeedback in the treatment of faecal incontinence. Biofeedback Self Regul 1984; 9: 311-324

17. Miner PB, Donelly TC, Read NW. Investigation of the mode of action of biofeedback in treatment of faecal incontinence. Dig Dis Sci 1990; 35: 1291-1298

18. Arhan P, Faverdin C, Devroede G et al. Biofeedback re-education of faecal continence in children. Int J Colorectal Dis 1994; 9: 128-133

19. Sangwan YP, Coller JA, Barrett RC, Roberts PL, Murray JJ, Schoetz DJ. Can manometric parameters predict response to biofeedback therapy in faecal incontinence? Dis Colon Rectum 1995; 38: 1021-1025

20. Glia A, Gylin M, Akerlund JE, Lindfors U, Lindberg G. Biofeedback training in patients with faecal incontinence. Dis Colon Rectum 1998; 41: 359-364

21. Fynes MM, Marshall K, Cassidy M et al. A prospective, randomised study comparing the effect of augmented biofeedback with sensory biofeedback alone on faecal incontinence after obstetric trauma. Dis Colon Rectum 1999; 42: 753-761

22. Whitehead WE, Engel BT, Schuster MM. Perception of rectal distension is necessary to prevent faecal incontinence. Adv Physiol Sci 1980; 17: 201-209

23. Wald A. Biofeedback for neurogenic faecal incontinence. Rectal sensation is a determinant of outcome. J Paediatr Gastroenterol Nutr 1983; 2: 302-306

24. McKee RF, McEnroe L, Anderson JH, Finlay IG. Identification of patients likely to benefit from biofeedback for outlet obstruction constipation. Br J Surg 1999; 86: 355-359

25. Chiotakakou-Faliakou E, Kamm MA, Roy AJ, Storrie JB, Turner IC. Biofeedback provides long term benefit for patients with intractable, slow transit constipation. Gut 1998; 42: 517-521

26. Bleijenberg G, Kuijpers HC. Treatment of the spastic pelvic floor syndrome with biofeedback. Dis Colon Rectum 1987; 30: 108-111

27. Shorvon PJ, McHugh S, Diamant NE, Somers S, Stevenson GW. Defaecography in normal volunteers: results and implications. Gut 1989; 30: 1737-1749

28. Voderholzer WA, Neuhaus DA, Klauser AG, Tzavella K, Muller-Lissner SA, Schindlbeck NE. Paradoxical sphincter contraction is rarely indicative of anismus. Gut 1997; 41: 258-262

29. Gilliland R, Heyman S, Altomare DF, Park UC, Vickers D, Wexner SD. Outcome and predictors of success of biofeedback for constipation. Br J Surg 1997; 84: 1123-1126

30. Gattuso J, Kamm MA. The management of constipation in adults. Ailment Pharmacol Ther 1993; 7: 487-500

31. Leroi AM, Duval V, Roussingnol C, Berkelmans I, Peninque P, Denis P. Biofeedback for anismus in 15 sexually abused women. Int J Colorectal Dis 1996; 11: 187-190

32. Drossman, D. The link between early abuse and GI disorders in women. Emergency Med 1992; 24 (6): 1-5

33. Keck JO, Staniunas RJ, Coller JA et al. Biofeedback training is useful in faecal incontinence but disappointing in constipation. Dis Colon Rectum 1994; 37: 1271-1276

34. Emmanuel AV, Kamm MA. Successful response to biofeedback for constipation is associated with specifically improved extrinsic autonomic innervation to the large bowel. Gastroenterology 1997; 112(suppl): A729 (abstract)

35. Azrin N, Foxx R. A rapid method of toilet training the institutionalised retarded. J Appl Behav Anal 1971; 4: 89-99

36. Pfeifer J, Agachan F, Wexner SD. Surgery for constipation: a review. Dis Colon Rectum 1996; 39: 444-460

37. Bernini A, Madoff RD, Lowry AC et al. Should patients with combined colonic inertia and nonrelaxing pelvic floor undergo subtotal colectomy? Dis Colon Rectum 1998; 41: 1363-1366

38. Devroede G. Constipation – a sign of a disease to be treated surgically or a symptom to be deciphered as nonverbal communication? (Editorial) J Clin Gastroenterol 1992; 15: 189-191

39. Barnes PRH, Gawley PR, Preston DM, Lennard-Jones JE. Experience of posterior division of the puborectalis muscle in the management of chronic constipation. Br J Surg 1985; 72: 475-477

40. Pinho M, Yoshioka K, Keighley MRB. Long-term results of anorectal myectomy for chronic constipation. Dis Colon Rectum 1990; 33: 795-797

41. Guthrie E, Creed F, Dawson D, Torrenson B. A controlled trial of psychological treatment for the irritable bowel syndrome. Gastroenterology 1991; 100: 450-457

42. Wise TN, Cooper JN, Ahmed S. The efficacy of group therapy for patients with IBS. Psychosomatics 1982; 23: 465

43. Dolk A, Holmstrom B, Johansson C, Frostell C, Nilsson BY. The effect of yoga on puborectalis paradox. Int J Colorectal Dis 1991; 6: 139-142

44. Karlbom U, Wattchow DA, Sarre RG et al. Prospective study of biofeedback for treatment of constipation. Dis Colon Rectum 1997; 40: 1143–1148

45. Mollen RMHG, Salvioli B, Camilleri M et al. The effects of biofeedback on rectal sensation and distal colonic motility in patients with disorders of rectal evacuation. Am J Gastroenterol 1999; 94: 751–756

46. Leahy A, Clayman C, Mason I, Lloyd G, Epstein O. Computerised biofeedback games: a new method for teaching stress management and its use in irritable bowel syndrome. J R Coll Physicians London 1998; 32: 552–556

47. Vaizey CJ, Roy AJ, Kamm MA. Prospective evaluation of the treatment of solitary rectal ulcer syndrome with biofeedback. Gut 1997; 41: 817–820

48. Arhan P, Faverdia C, Devroede G et al. Biofeedback re-education of faecal incontinence in children. Int J Colorectal Dis 1994; 9: 128–133

49. Whitehead WE, Burgio KL, Engel BT. Biofeedback treatment of faecal incontinence in geriatric patients. J Am Geriatr Soc 1985; 33: 320–324

50. Stanley R. Treatment of continence in people with learning disabilities: 3. Br J Nursing 1997; 6: 12–22

Chapter 10
Developing methods in physiological assessment

DAVID F EVANS AND ETSURO YAZAKI

Physiological assessment of the gastrointestinal (GI) tract has become an essential tool in the diagnosis of many digestive diseases. Over the last century, scientific breakthroughs, such as the discovery of peristalsis by Bayliss and Starling[1] and the existence of an independent 'brain in the gut'[2], have set the scene for recent innovations for assessment of the physiology and pathophysiology of gut function. The whole area of measurement of function has been hindered in the past because the gut is a relatively inaccessible organ. In addition to this, it has been realized that measurements need to be made over long periods, as a result of the nature of the periodicity of normal gut function.

Many techniques are new and development has had to await significant technical inventions and advances. With the invention of sophisticated transducers and recording instrumentation, particularly with the introduction of microchip technology, there have been considerable advances in the ability to investigate most parts of the human GI tract. This chapter discusses those areas that remain under development and have potential for incorporation into the currently available techniques.

Clinical need

The requirement to develop new techniques to investigate the GI tract has arisen for a number of reasons. First, gastroenterology has been an area of medicine that has seriously lagged behind other specialities in terms of fundamental knowledge relating to normal function. Second, there has appeared to be a dramatic increase in the incidence of chronic, non-life-threatening, gastrointestinal disorders, particularly in Western societies, and this has also driven the development of existing technology. Third, in this day and age, patients are more health conscious and are unwilling to tolerate niggling digestive problems, such as dyspepsia, and again this has driven the requirement for objective demonstrations of dysfunction in order to treat such conditions more effectively.

This chapter illustrates some of the more important new investigations that are under development or in current use in specialist centres.

Developing methodology

Imaging and transit

These techniques involve the production of visual images from within the body. The digestive tract is well suited to these techniques because most parts of the gut are totally inaccessible as a result of its length and position, deep in the abdominal cavity.

Impedance

Three specific methods of detection of transit using impedance have been developed[3-5] and show promise. All rely on the principle that the GI tract acts as an electrically conducting hollow lumen lying within a conductive cavity, the abdomen.

Principle

The impedance of the gut lumen can be detected by passing a small alternating current across or within the gut wall and measuring the resultant voltage on the opposite surface or axially, either to construct images or to measure motor function. By filling the lumen with a substance of either greater or lower conductance than the viscera, a change in impedance can be detected. If the change in impedance over time is plotted, movement of luminal content can be detected from one area to another, i.e. gastric emptying, oesophageal transit, and rectal filling and emptying.

Methodology

Epigastrography

This system uses two electrodes per channel, usually with two channels. A current is passed anterior to posterior across the gastric region and a voltage plot drawn of the underlying resistance across the gastric lumen. Gastric filling and emptying of selected test meals (mainly liquids) are plotted as a change in impedance with a gradual return to baseline. The technique is highly sensitive to movement artefacts and gastric acid secretion, and has been mainly used in clinical trials of drugs affecting motor activity of the stomach.

Electrical impedance tomography

This technique produces a two-dimensional colour tomogram (similar to a computed tomography [CT] scan, but with less detail) of a 4- to 6-cm transverse section across the abdomen underlying 16 surface ECG-type electrodes positioned in a horizontal ring, usually overlying the stomach. Each electrode pair sequentially acts as a current generator and receiver, and the resultant impedance tomogram is plotted as a full-colour impedance 'contour' picture. Movement of luminal content can be plotted as impedance changes in the contour map. Quantification of data can be achieved by drawing regions of interest over specific areas and plotting luminal movement against time (Figure 10.1).

The technique has been researched in many areas of medicine, including cardiac, respiratory and neurological imaging. In gastroenterology, the technique has been developed mainly to image the stomach as an alternative to gamma scintigraphy in the assessment of gastric emptying. The technique is non-invasive and uses no ionizing radiation (X-rays, isotopes); it is therefore suitable for use in multiple examinations (e.g. clinical trials) or in those patients unsuitable for radiation (pregnancy, infants, children, etc.).

The technique is also sensitive to gastric acid and has been advocated as a non-invasive measure of acid secretion.[6] As a result of the acid sensitivity, it has been suggested that electrical impedance tomography may be a more physiological measurement of gastric function than other methods because it detects luminal volume, i.e. ingested food content plus secretions.[7]

Potential uses

Although the overall technique remains mainly in the research domain at present, it offers a safe, non-invasive method of measurement. It is ideal for patients who are not suitable for imaging with X-rays or isotopes, i.e. children and pregnant women, or individuals who require multiple measurements, e.g. in clinical trials of new drugs. The equipment is inexpensive and portable and does not require sophisticated professionals or expensive consumables. At present, research has concentrated on techniques

Feed

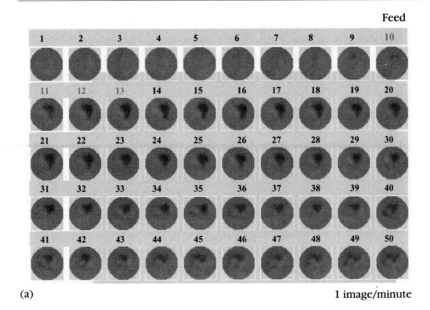

(a)   1 image/minute

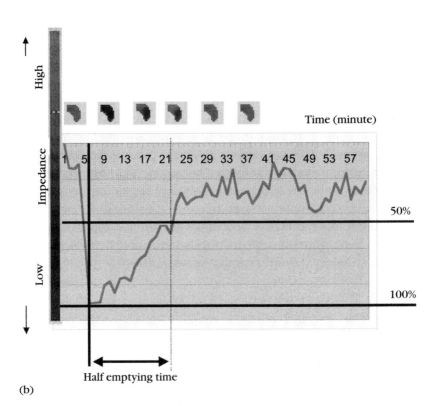

(b)

Figure 10.1 Electrical impedance tomography (a) and gastric emptying curve (b).

of gastric emptying, although the scope is limited only by the ingenuity of researchers in the field.

Impedancometry

This is a new technique, again using the principle of electrical impedance. The technique was developed in Germany[5, 8] and recently commercialized in the USA (Sandhill Scientific, Colorado).

It is advocated as an alternative method to manometry and Bilitec to simultaneously monitor oesophageal motility, and acid and non-acid reflux. The technique is currently being researched and may replace simple pH measurements in the assessment of the patient with reflux symptoms.

Principle

A small (2-mm diameter) polyvinyl catheter assembly houses 6–14 ring electrodes spaced in pairs over a 25-cm length, and also a single antimony, pH-sensitive electrode. The catheter is positioned nasally such that the pH sensor lies 5 cm above the lower oesophageal sphincter and the impedance electrodes straddle the length of the oesophagus. The catheter is connected to a signal conditioning unit and PC, and small electrical currents are passed simultaneously through the electrodes. Alterations in impedance are caused by swallowing normal foodstuffs and drinks, and by reflux of food or acidic gastric juice. Continuous traces are recorded digitally and can be analysed by dedicated software, although at present automated analysis is still in its infancy. Figure 10.2 illustrates a recording showing a swallow.

Potential uses

If the technique proves sensitive and specific, it could replace conventional methods of measurement. With the introduction of an ambulatory recorder and development of automated analysis, impedancometry may be a single-catheter alternative to prolonged manometry, pH and bile monitoring.

Fast magnetic resonance imaging

Principle

Conventional magnetic resonance imaging (MRI) is now widely used as an imaging technique in medical diagnostics but, as yet,

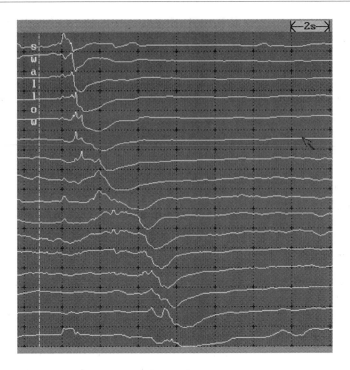

Figure 10.2 Impedancometry: swallow.

apart from its potential use in the staging of certain types of GI tumours, it has seen little development in gastroenterology. This is because conventional MRI requires long imaging times (seconds to minutes) to build up an acceptable picture as a result of the low energies produced by the magnetic resonance technique. This has meant that MRI has been suitable only for static, or non-moving, organs and has excluded imaging of organs undergoing periodic or aperiodic motion, such as the heart, lungs and viscera. Although gating has been used to help visualize some organs such as heart and lungs, these modifications do not help when imaging the GI tract. At best, fast low angle shot imaging (FLASH) has been used to assess gastric emptying[9].

Echo planar imaging (EPI) is a relatively new MR technique whereby a complete image can be produced in a fraction of a second, thus, for the first time, enabling pictures of aperiodic movement to be produced. The first reports of the use of echo planar imaging in the evaluation of upper gastrointestinal motility[10], and more recently with longer imaging periods of many hours[11], herald a new era in non-invasive investigation of the GI tract (Figure 10.3).

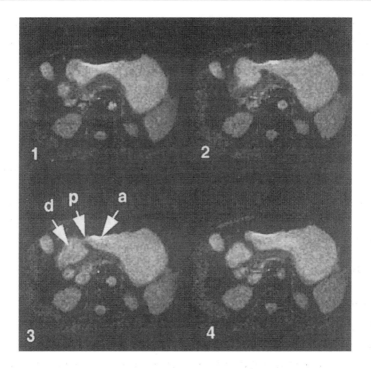

Figure 10.3 Fast magnetic resonance imaging.

Methodology

Echo planar imaging can be performed only using an MR scanner with special hardware and software, although it is now possible to 'add on' EPI hardware and software to conventional scanners and this will make it possible in the future to use the facilities of fast MRI in the general hospital setting.

Potential uses

With further research, MRI will increasingly be used more in the visual imaging of the upper GI tract and may in future replace radiology in some areas.

Motor function and visceral sensitivity

Prolonged manometry

The measurement of motility in the upper GI tract, including functional studies of the oesophagus, stomach and small intestine, has become of increasing interest to gastro-enterologists in recent years. Motility of the gut smooth muscle is controlled by the myenteric plexus and is responsible for the mixing, direction, velocity and flow of intraluminal content. This is important because it is now thought that defects in normal motility are responsible for many of the functional bowel disorders currently recognized.[12] Manometry uses the technique of detection of gut wall contractions by intraluminal pressure sensors mounted on catheters that are passed into the gut lumen. With two or more sensors, the differences between propulsive and non-propulsive contractions can be recognized. Conventional manometry has been available for many years; more recently, with the development of powerful portable recording devices, this technique can be performed for long periods under ambulatory conditions.

Techniques

Strain gauge microtransducers

Miniature strain gauges mounted on a fine flexible catheter are essential in the measurement of GI motility in ambulatory patients.

Electrical strain gauges deform when a positive or negative pressure is applied to the surface. In the gut, the deformation is generally produced by contracting smooth muscle (and corresponding gut wall movement), but a pressure rise in the lumen is required to alter the electrical output. In organs with a large viscus (e.g. gastric fundus, rectum) other techniques may be more representative of motor function, such as the barostat (see below). Although expensive (£500–£1000 per channel), strain gauges obviate the need for water perfusion and can be used more easily in the ambulatory mode[13].

Recorders

In recent years, gastroenterologists have recognized that the symptoms of disordered GI function are often intermittent and that representative measurements may be better obtained by prolonged recordings. Furthermore, circadian changes in gut biorhythms require that measurements are made to span a normal daily cycle, i.e. in most cases for a minimum of 24 hours. This requirement, together with the rapid development in computer technology, has seen the introduction of digital recording systems; these have sufficient memory capacity and on-board computer processing power to allow high-fidelity recordings from multi-channel sensors for long periods, in some cases over many days. Equipment is battery powered, light and portable, and allows for almost total ambulation during measurement. This means not only that recordings are made in near-physiological conditions, but also that patients can undergo measurements in their homes and workplaces. Event markers also allow for correlation between patients' symptoms and abnormalities in the measured parameter.

The addition of such technology has also added the ability to analyse recordings with sophisticated computer software programs – a further benefit of both savings in time and the rapid acquisition of accurate, repeatable, unbiased information derived from large quantities of data[14].

Potential uses

Oesophagus

Ambulatory manometry of the oesophagus is becoming an established technique for the investigation of symptoms of non-cardiac chest pain, and other symptoms thought to be of oesophageal origin undiagnosed by conventional manometry or pH monitoring. The technique has been well researched[15, 16] and is fast becoming one of the options available to GI physiologists in the clinical investigation units. With semi-automated analysis and transducers that will measure sphincter and body motility, patients with hitherto undiagnosed, intermittent symptoms can now be diagnosed and treatment-optimized using the new technologies.

Sphincter of Oddi

Sphincter of Oddi manometry has been advocated in the assessment of sphincter of Oddi dysfunction. The technique is generally performed during endoscopic examination of the biliary tree (endoscopic retrograde cholangiopancreatography [ERCP]), and currently is unphysiological and allows for only short-term assessment[17]. New techniques under development may allow for more prolonged studies, with the possibility in the future for ambulatory studies using an indwelling transducer in the bile or pancreatic ducts[18]. Modern fibreoptic technology will provide micropressure transducers (0.1-mm diameter) which can be placed at ERCP and left *in situ*. Only then will it be possible to assess intermittent dysfunction in the sphincter of Oddi.

Small intestine

Failure of the small intestine is a life-threatening group of diseases caused by loss of effective motility and digestive and absorptive capacity in the bowel. Currently, treatment consists of either long-term parenteral nutrition or transplantation, both having high morbidity and mortality rates. Symptoms of small intestinal dysfunction can be confused with less serious conditions of visceral hypersensitivity (irritable bowel syndrome, painless diarrhoea, non-ulcer dyspepsia) and any investigation that helps to differentiate the two conditions is clearly of benefit.

Prolonged, ambulatory small intestinal manometry of the proximal small intestine identifies normal fasting and postprandial motor patterns, as well as differences in circadian patterns[19]. With the advent of computer analysis[20], it is now possible to identify the onset of the abnormal motor activity that is associated with small intestinal motor diseases (pseudo-obstruction, enteral neuropathy/myopathy).

The technique involves the passage of a long, multi-channel, strain-gauge catheter into the jejunum and monitoring patients during normal activities over a 24-hour period. The recording is analysed for motor activity during and after a meal and at night. Frequency plots can show the results of loss of myenteric plexus control and the pathology associated with small intestine dys-function (Figure 10.4).

This is another technique that has predominantly been used only for research, but with further development it will be used as a standard clinical tool in some centres within the next few years

Colon and rectum

Our knowledge of normal physiological function of the mechanisms responsible for defecation has led to this area of investigation being the second most widely available GI function technique in medical and surgical gastroenterology departments. By contrast, the paucity of information about colonic and rectal function has led to a reduced interest in this area, even though there are many common lower GI disorders that are undoubtedly caused by motor dysfunction of the colon and rectum, e.g. two of the most common manifestations of colorectal dysfunction are constipation and diarrhoea. The two opposing conditions relating to either slow or rapid transit of colonic contents are poorly understood in relation to the physiology of the large bowel; the pathophysiology of the disorders is understood even less. The reasons for this are complex, but part of the problem is the difficulty in the past of measuring motor function of the colon over prolonged periods.

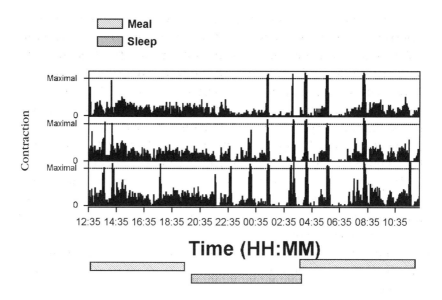

Figure 10.4a 24-hour frequency plot of small intestinal motility from a normal volunteer.

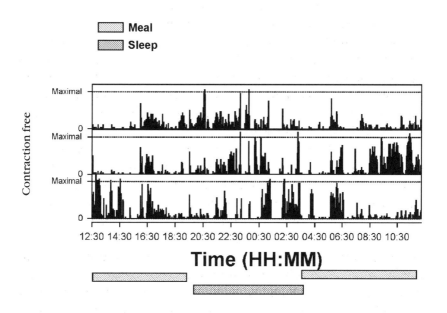

Figure 10.4b 24 hour frequency plots obtained from a patient with pseudo obstruction.

Manometry has previously been studied by insertion of catheters housing pressure sensors into the prepared colon at flexible colonoscopy. This has yielded some information but has not really advanced our understanding of colonic function because of difficulties in obtaining and interpretation of data[21]. Now, with the increased availability of multi-channel recorders and catheters, and the advances in placement of the catheters without prior bowel preparation, there has been a resurgence of interest in this area and a few centres have started to investigate the field again. Recently, using such technology[22], new information relating to the way in which the colon handles undigested fats and carbohydrates is giving us important clues as to the nature of functional bowel diseases and their relationship to diet.

No doubt in future, as more centres use the new technologies, colorectal manometry will become useful in the diagnosis of colonic disorders.

Barostat (visceral stimulator)

Principle

The barostat is a device that measures compliance of the stomach and other visci with a significant volume, such as the rectum. The device consists of two major components: a non-compliant balloon, which can be inserted into the organ and be continuously inflated and deflated by an external pump, and a pressure-sensing device that monitors the pressure within the balloon. The two systems are linked such that either can control the other, i.e. constant pressure with variable volume, or constant volume with varying pressure[23].

By varying the inflation pressures and volumes to fixed levels, the device can be used to test the sensitivity of the organ under examination; e.g. where rectal hypersensitivity is suspected in a patient with either urgency of defecation or an 'irritable bowel', the balloon can be inflated to different volumes or pressures to test for increased hypersensitivity of the rectal wall. This can be useful in determining the nature of the disease and how best to treat it. In the stomach this technique has been used to investigate non-ulcer dyspepsia[24], and with the introduction of commercially available equipment, more techniques are likely to follow in future years.

Methodology

The patient is intubated with a multi-lumen polyvinyl catheter, which consists of a minimum of two recording channels and incorporates a thin, non-compliant balloon of varying capacity depending on the target organ. The balloon is positioned in the target organ and the assembly connected to the barostat control unit. The study protocol is dictated by the clinical question but, by controlling either volume or pressure, compliance (elasticity) of the wall of the organ can be assessed (fixed pressure), or wall sensitivity to distension can be assessed by keeping the volume constant and increasing the pressure.

Potential clinical uses

Oesophagus

In the oesophagus, the barostat is being used to research its potential in assessment of swallowing disorders where a possible cause is related to stiffened upper or lower sphincters, either from an idiopathic cause or by damage from refluxed acid or bile (strictures)[25].

Stomach

In the stomach, the barostat is being used to investigate the possible role of gastric wall stiffening in relation to non-ulcer dyspepsia, bloating, early satiety, nausea and even idiopathic vomiting. In this case, the relationship to symptoms is assessed by measuring the pressure–volume curves generated by the receptive relaxation of the gastric fundus as a result of distension. This has been shown to be altered in some patients with dyspepsia[25].

Rectum

The barostat has also been used in the rectum to assess patients with defecatory disorders. In this case, rectal compliance is used as a measure of rectal sensitivity. Where sensitivity is low, patients may be constipated and may not detect the normal call to stool when the rectum is full. Where sensitivity is high, rectal filling may be far from complete when the desire to defecate is sensed. In this area of medicine, this sort of information may be extremely useful in the treatment of 'functional' and organic evacuatory diseases[26].

Non-acid reflux

There is an increasing interest in the investigation of 'non-acid' or bile reflux. This is related to the potential association of biliary reflux as a carcinogen in the development of cancer of the gastro-oesophageal junction.

During the past 10 or so years, there is increasing evidence that a mixture of acid and bile reflux may be a potent agent in the development of Barrett's oesophagus[27]. This is a condition whereby the normal oesophageal squamous epithelium is replaced by gastric-type columnar cells and it is these cells that undergo metaplasia and dysplasia, and terminate in carcinoma *in situ*. The disease is increasing at an alarming rate and therefore there has been a desire to measure the presence of both oesophageal and gastric bile reflux.

Many methods have been advocated but all previous attempts have limitations. A new technique with some promise is now available commercially.

Bilitec

Principle

The Bilitec is a portable ambulatory recording system that uses a spectrophotometric principle, whereby the absorption of the substance bilirubin (the pigmented chemical found in bile) is detected with an infrared probe positioned in the distal oesophagus or stomach. The presence of bilirubin signifies the presence of bile and this, together with other corrosive gastric fluids, may be relevant to the progression of reflux disease, through Barrett's oesophagus, into carcinoma.

Methodology

A catheter of specialized design, incorporating an infrared photometric sensor at its tip is connected to a purpose-built, portable digital recorder, which is carried by the patient. The probe is positioned in the distal oesophagus or stomach and detects bile reflux; it can be used to pinpoint some of the symptoms in patients with gastro-oesophageal reflux disease (GORD) that may be caused by bile reflux and not just acid alone. Prolonged ambulatory measurements are usually carried out in conjunction with oesophageal pH, and patients are encouraged to eat and drink normally. As the bilirubin sensor is also sensitive to dark-coloured foods, these need to be avoided during measurements to prevent false-positive results. Published works using this technique have established normal values[28] and examined bilirubin levels in complicated GORD patients[29].

Figure 10.5 shows two 24-hour records of normal and abnormal recordings.

Potential uses

This investigation can help in the diagnosis of non-acid reflux in patients with systems that are difficult to treat, or help to guide the clinician to alter treatments where high levels of alkaline reflux may require surgical correction.

Electrogastrography

Principle

The electrical rhythm of the upper GI tract can be detected by placing sensing electrodes intraluminally, serosally or on the skin surface overlying the organ of interest. In humans, the intraluminal and skin surface methods are the two most practical techniques and most studies to date have concentrated on electrical activity emanating from the stomach; this technique is called electro-gastrography (EGG)[30]. The EGG in humans runs at a basal rate of 3 counts/min and has been shown to alter in amplitude during feeding and frequency in pathological conditions, such as idiopathic vomiting and non-ulcer dyspepsia[31, 32]. There may also be a possibility that, with suitable signal processing, the indirect detection of motility may be possible.

Electrogastrography, as with other new methods, is mainly driven by available technology and, with the recent introduction of a commercially available portable EGG recorder, more research is bound to follow. The technique is very attractive as a possible alternative to tube methods of motility measurement, especially in patient groups where intubation may be undesirable, e.g. in children[33].

Methodology

Two standard disposable ECG, surface electrodes are attached to the skin overlying the gastric body and antrum. The position is usually straddling the midline and about a third of the distance between the umbilicus and the navel. A third electrode is placed

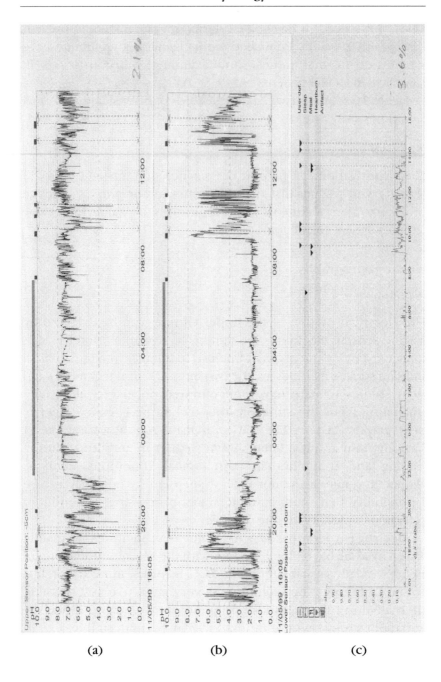

(a)   (b)   (c)

Figure 10.5a Normal dual-channel (oesophagus (a) and gastric (b)) 24-hour pH recordings and normal oesophageal Bilitec (c) recordings, obtained simultaneously.

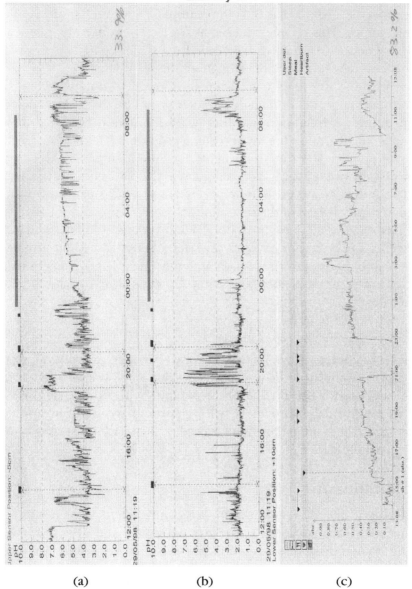

(a)   (b)   (c)

Figure 10.5b 24-hour dual-channel pH recordings showing abnormal acid GOR (a), normal gastric (b) and abnormal levels of oesophageal bile (c).

over a bony area, usually the xiphisternum, and this acts as a reference earth. The electrodes are connected to a purpose-built, portable, digital datalogger (Medtronic Ltd), using a special connector lead that has built-in preamplifiers for each of the active electrodes. This reduces the signal artefacts produced by physical movement. EGG signals are recorded at 1 Hz for up to 24 hours and patients may be ambulant throughout the recordings.

Various protocols have been developed to obtain the most representative recordings. One such protocol[33] has a formalized structure. A baseline recording of 15 minutes is followed by a standard meal and a further recording of 2 hours. This is rather rigid in approach; other methods allow for complete patient freedom with unrestricted meals and activities, and a full 24-hour recording. The latter, however, is more prone to artefacts caused by the ambulatory nature of the recordings.

Normal values have been obtained in various groups[34, 35] and the scene is now set for examining various potential patient groups. Possible targets are those patients with unexplained, functional, foregut symptoms such as dyspepsia, nausea, early satiety and bloating.

Potential uses

If clear differences can be demonstrated between various symptom groups, ambulatory EGG will be a useful, non-invasive screening procedure for the evaluation of patients with functional upper gastrointestinal disorders. It will be particularly useful in patient groups where the non-invasive nature of the test is most attractive, e.g. children.

Conclusion

It is clear that, during the technological revolution of the last three decades, new advances in sensors, hardware and software have led to exciting new possibilities in the investigation of the gastrointestinal tract. This, together with an increasing knowledge of the physiology and pathophysiology of GI tract function, will lead to better treatments of hitherto under-diagnosed and poorly treated symptoms caused by functional bowel disorders. In the future, it may be possible for the physician, as depicted in sci-fi stories, to 'strap on' a machine that will give a rapid diagnosis of the underlying disorder – Dr McCoy of Star Trek fame may not be as far away as we think!

References

1. Bayliss WM, Starling EH. The movements and innervation of the small intestine. J Physiol 1899; 24: 99–143
2. Wingate DL. Backwards and forwards with the migrating motor complex. Am J Dig Dis 1981; 26: 641–666
3. Sutton JA, Thompson S, Sobnack R. Measurement of gastric emptying rates by radioactive isotope scanning and epigastric impedance. Lancet 1985; ii: 898–890
4. Brown BH. Tissue impedance methods. In: Jackson DF (ed.), Imaging of Non-ionising Radiations. Guildford: Surrey University Press: 83–110
5. Silny J. Intraluminal multiple impedance procedure for measurement of gastrointestinal motility. J Gastroint Motility 1991; 3: 151–162
6. Baxter AJ, Mangnall YF, Loj EJ et al. Evaluation of applied potential tomography as a new non-invasive test of gastric secretion. Gut 1988; 29: 1730
7. Wright JW, Evans DF, Bush D, Ledingham SJ. The effect of nutrient and non-nutrient test meals on gastric emptying using EIT. In: Holder D (ed.), Clinical and Physiological Applications of Electric Impedance Tomography. London: UCL Press, 1993:100
8. Sifrim D, Silny J, Holloway RH, Janssens JJ. Patterns of gas and liquid reflux during transient relaxations of the lower oesophageal sphincter: a study using intraluminal electrical impedance. Gut 1999; 44: 47–54
9. Schwizer W, Maeke M, Fried M. Measurement of gastric emptying by magnetic resonance imaging in humans. Gastroenterology 1992; 103: 369
10. Stehling MK, Evans DF, Lamont G et al. Gastrointestinal tract: dynamic MR studies using echo-planar imaging. Radiology 1989; 171: 41
11. Evans DF, Lamont GL, Stehling MK et al. Prolonged monitoring of the upper gastrointestinal tract using echo-planar magnetic resonance imaging. Gut 1993; 34: 848–852
12. Stacher G. Motor disorders of the stomach and duodenum. In: Kumar D, Wingate DL (eds), An Illustrated Guide to Gastrointestinal Motility, 2nd edn. London: Churchill Livingstone, 1993: 522
13. Gill RC, Kellow JE, Browning C, Wingate DL. The use of intraluminal strain gauges for recording ambulant small bowel motility. Am J Physiol 1990; 258: G610
14. Castillo FD, Benson MJ, Wingate DL, Samaras T, Spyrou NM. Evaluation of computerised analysis of propagation of human duodenjejunal contractions. J Neurogastroenterol Motility 1994; 6: 11
15. Barham CP, Gotley DC, Miller R, Mills A, Alderson D. Ambulatory measurement of oesophageal function: clinical use of a new pH and motility recording system. Br J Surg 1992; 79: 1056
16. Bremner RM, Constantini M, DeMeester TR et al. Normal oesophageal body function: a study using ambulatory oesophageal manometry. Am J Gastroenterol 1997; 42: 183–187
17. Toouli J, Craig A. Sphincter of Oddi function and dysfunction. Can J Gastroenterol 2000; 14: 411–419
18. Wehrmann T, Schmitt T, Schonfield A, Caspary WF, Seifert H. Endoscopic sphincter of Oddi manometry with a portable electronic microtransducer system: comparison with the perfusion manometry method. Endoscopy 2000; 32: 444–451
19. Fell JM, Smith VV, Milla PJ. Infantile chronic intestinal pseudo-obstruction: the role of small intestinal manometry. Gut 1996; 39: 306–311

20. Benson MJ, Castillo FD, Wingate DL, Spyrou NM. The computer as referee in the analysis of human small bowel motility. Am J Physiol 1993; 264: G645-G665

21. Narducci F, Bassotti G, Gaburri M, Morelli A. Twenty four hour manometric recording of colonic motor activity in healthy man. Gut 1987; 28: 17-25

22. Rao SS, Kavelock R, Beaty J, Ackerson K, Stumbo P. Effects of fat and carbohydrate meals on colonic motor response. Gut 1999; 46: 205-211

23. Azpiroz F, Malagelada JR. Physiological variations in canine gastric tone measured by an electronic barostat. Am J Physiol 1985; 248: G229

24. Salet G, Sansom M, Roelofs JM, van Berge Henegouwen GP, Smout AJ, Akkermans LM. Response to gastric distension in functional dyspepsia. Gut 1998; 42: 823-829

25. Gonzales M, Mearin F, Vasconez C, Armengol JR, Malagelada JR. Oesophageal tone in patients with achalasia. Gut 1997; 41: 291-296

26. Leroi AM, Saiter C, Roussignol C, Weber J, Denis P. Increased tone of the rectal wall in response to feeding persists in patients with cauda equina syndrome. Neurogastroenterol Motility 1999; 11: 243-245

27. Vaezi MF, Richter JE. Bile reflux in columnar lined oesophagus. Gastroenterol Clinics North Am 1997; 26: 565-582

28. Byrne JP, Romagnoli R, Bechi P, Fuchs K, Collard JM. Duodenogastric reflux of bile in health: normal range. Physiological Measurement 1999; 20: 149-158

29. Marshall RE, Anggiansah A, Manifold D, Owen WJ. Effect of omeprazole 20mg twice daily on duodenogastric and gastro-oesophageal bile reflux in Barrett's oesophagus. Gut 1998; 43: 603-606

30. Stern RM. A brief history of the electrogastrogram. In: Stern RM, Koch KL (eds), Electrogastrography: Methodology, Techniques and Validation. New York: Praeger, 1985: 3

31. Geldhof H, Van der Schee EJ, van Blankenstein M, Grashuis JL. Electro-gastrographic study of gastric myoelectrical activity in patients with unexplained nausea and vomiting. Gut 1986; 27: 799

32. Familioni BO, Bowes KL, Kingma YJ, Cote KR. Can transcutaneous recordings detect gastric electrical abnormalities? Gut 1991; 32: 141

33. Milla PJ. Electrogastrography in children: an overview. In: Chen JZ, McCallum RW (eds), Electrogastrography: Principles and Applications. New York: Raven Press, 1994: 379

34. Riezzi G, Chiloiro M, Guerra V, Borrelli O, Salvia G, Cuchiarra S. Comparison of gastric electrical activity and gastric emptying in healthy and dyspeptic children. Dig Dis Sci 2000; 45: 517-524

35. Leahy A, Besherdas K, Clayman C, Mason I, Epstein O. Abnormalities of the electrogastrogram in functional gastrointestinal disorders. Am J Gastroenterol 1999; 94: 1023-1028

Chapter 11

The role of the nurse practitioner in clinical physiology

Spike Smilgin Humphreys

Since Kronecher and Meltzer[1] first described oesophageal manometry in 1883, measurement of gastrointestinal (GI) motility has been largely conducted by academic clinicians or scientists, assisted in many cases by laboratory technicians. The presence of nurses in any capacity other than as doctors' attendants would have been very unlikely in the early days of investigations. In the latter part of the twentieth century, manometry studies as we know them today were developed to investigate motor function and, as computer technology opened the field even further, gastro-enterologists, GI surgeons and clinical scientists began to work more closely together to develop the speciality of GI clinical measurement. Some nurses were attracted to this discipline, invited by enlightened clinicians recognizing that the presence of a nurse would be an asset in the physiology laboratory. This action was considered by some nursing colleagues to fly in the face of tradition; fears were voiced that nurses were turning their backs on the essence of nursing and that taking an interest in machinery and computers precluded caring for patients to the standard demanded by their training.

Inevitably nurses, who were concerned with holistic care of the patient and may have worked previously on the periphery of investigation laboratories, began to take more interest in the work of the laboratory itself. They recognized that where there was a patient there was a place for nursing skills, in conjunction with conducting actual investigations. Thus came the advent of the GI clinical measurement nurse practitioner (this term is not recognized by the United Kingdom Central Council for Nursing, Midwifery and Health Visiting [UKCC], as all nurses are practitioners in their own right[2]), clinical nurse specialist in GI physiology, nurse physiologist and nurse clinician. This point is expounded by Finlay[3]. The work is still in its relative infancy and therefore an agreed title has yet to be established, each unit preferring to use the description that suits its particular purpose. Standardization will inevitably occur along with desired academic requirements and ultimately official recognition. Until then, we are in the privileged position of developing this exciting new area of care. For the purposes of this chapter, this role is referred to as nurse physiologist.

The publication of *The Scope of Professional Practice*[4] - a UKCC position statement outlining the scope of professional practice – gave further confidence to nurses who may otherwise have felt out of their depth in a potentially alien field or who experienced some confusion between the essential nursing role and that of the technologist. It recognizes the developing role of nursing practice, stating that:

> Practice takes place in a context of continuing change and development. Such change and development may result from advances in research leading to improvements in treatment and care, from alterations to the provision of health and social care services, as a result of changes in local policies and as a result of new approaches to professional practice. Practice must, therefore, be sensitive, relevant and responsive to the needs of individual patients and clients and have the capacity to adjust, where and when appropriate, to changing circumstances.

Personnel

Who are the people who take up GI clinical measurement as a career? Do they undertake this work because they are interested in basic/advanced science, which is the lynchpin of the work, or because they are interested in the individuals on whom the measurements are carried out? The answer is probably that scientists/technicians are, on the whole, motivated by the former and nurses by the latter. GI physiology departments are mostly run by clinical scientists who have degrees and doctorates in their subject, who have undertaken a great deal of research on the way and who have now taken on the running of the department, a task not only requiring intimate knowledge of the subject, but also good management skills. The motivation for their work is likely to be the furtherance of understanding of the science involved. Technicians, or medical technical officers, are usually young people with an interest in science and basic qualifications who may have an ambition to become a clinical scientist. To establish a career in GI science these officers are required to gain qualifications in medical physics and physiological measurement. Undoubtedly patient management is addressed during the period of training, but constraints of time and resources would preclude this from being much more than cursory. In multidisciplinary departments, however, this situation is addressed on a daily basis, with scientists learning nursing skills from the professionals. At the same time, nurses are able to increase their body of knowledge from their scientist colleagues. This philosophy is advocated by the UKCC[5], which states that:

> As a registered nurse, midwife or health visitor, you are personally accountable for your practice and, in the exercise of your professional accountability must . . .

> 6 work in a collaborative and co-operative manner with health care professionals and others involved in providing care, and recognise and respect their particular contributions within the care team; . . .

> 14 assist professional colleagues, in the context of your own knowledge, experience and sphere of responsibility, to develop their professional competence and assist others in the care team, including informal carers, to contribute safely to a degree appropriate to their roles.

It is not feasible to be all things to all people.

Nurse physiologists are likely to be specialists coming from a variety of backgrounds, including gastroenterology wards, endoscopy, stomatherapy, operating theatres and outpatients, and will have had some years of post-registration experience in their field. They will have spent much time acquiring teaching, counselling and management expertise, and will have become proficient in budget management, audit, infection control and communication skills – all essential requirements for successful management of a GI physiology department – in addition to understanding the technology. A nurse's particular training in caring for the individual in a holistic manner (defined as emphasizing the importance of the whole and the interdependence of its parts) will undoubtedly be of benefit to patients undergoing investigations. Until the raging debate about titles reaches resolution, nurses experienced in managing GI physiology departments should probably be described as advanced nurse practitioners[3]. An experienced nurse with ingrained and well-practised concern for the welfare of patients and an interest in technology would enjoy the challenge of combining these skills, never forgetting the *raison d'être* of a nurse, which is to care for patients. The challenge is to bring about a situation where both disciplines converge and work together to create an environment in which people who present with symptoms of disordered motility can have their problems investigated in a place where they feel safe and comfortable – where they will not have their dignity compromised and can gain information about their condition, thus going forward towards treatment fully informed.

Investigations

Gastrointestinal clinical measurement is discussed in greater depth in other chapters in this book, but the investigations can be essentially divided into upper- and lower-tract studies:

A1   Investigations into the physiology of the upper intestinal tract concern measurement of pH, when the level of acid refluxing from the stomach into the oesophagus is assessed over a period of 24 hours. The patient is required to attend the physiology unit for the intranasal insertion of the manometry catheter into the oesophagus, and then to go home and carry on life as normally as possible, returning 24 hours later for the catheter and its recording device to be removed and the recorded data to be downloaded into the computer for analysis.

A2   Oesophageal motility studies examine muscular activity in the oesophagus and its upper and lower sphincters in patients who complain of dysphagia or who have pain or discomfort in the throat, chest or epigastrium. These tests can be stationary – conducted in the unit for a period lasting anything from 10 minutes to over an hour – or ambulatory – where, once again, the patient is required to go home for 24 hours wearing an intranasal manometry catheter, attached to a recording device worn over the shoulder or around the waist, returning the following day for removal of the equipment and analysis of the data. Indeed, the shorter version of these investigations is required before acid reflux can be measured, so that the manometry catheter may be positioned correctly, its tip at 5 cm above the proximal end of the lower oesophageal sphincter (LOS) (see Chapter 3).

A1 and A2 are the most commonly conducted investigations. Others concern measurement of bile reflux, gastric emptying, hydrogen breath tests, close examination of the upper oesophageal sphincter (UOS) and certain provocation tests.

B1   Lower GI physiology investigations include a number of highly specialized motility assessments. Those carried out most specifically at John Radcliffe Hospital, Oxford, concern measurement of structures in the pelvic floor, namely pressure and sensation recordings in the anal canal and rectum, and anal endosonography (see Chapters 6 and 8). Conditions requiring such investigations include:
- congenital disorders
- smooth muscle disorders
- Crohn's disease and colitis
- diarrhoea
- constipation/evacuation difficulties
- incontinence
- fissure/fistula *in ano*
- Hirschsprung's disease
- mucosal/rectal prolapse
- megarectum
- neosphincter
- neurological disorder
- pre-/post-anal/rectal surgery
- proctalgia fugax
- post-spinal injury/surgery
- post-obstetric trauma
- rectocele
- radiation proctitis
- solitary rectal ulcer

(see Chapter 5).

B2   Pelvic floor therapies such as biofeedback (see Chapter 9) have been implemented in the treatment of both faecal incontinence and constipation.

Although nursing skills are undisputedly of benefit when conducting any GI physiology investigation, they are particularly crucial when investigating colonic or anorectal disorders. In our culture many people are reluctant to discuss disorders of the pelvic floor (although more so with anorectal rather than urogynaecological disorders). In particular, some of the older generation have been brought up to believe not only that this area is especially 'private' but also that it is sometimes 'dirty', and that they must be perverse even to consider seeking help to address whatever the problem may be, instead of just putting up with it or managing it themselves at home. This natural reticence makes it very difficult to establish the percentage of the population who have pelvic floor disorders, because it is very likely that most people just put up with the situation. Therefore people who actually reach investigation units in hospitals must be the 'tip of the iceberg' and must be managed with great delicacy. On the other hand, many patients, again mostly older ones, still believe that hospitals are staffed with people of god-like status and they must abandon themselves to the will and whims of the experts, rather than adopting a more proactive stance with their own bodies. Nursing skills really come into play here: welcoming patients into the department, encouraging them to participate in the investigations of their own free will, and being reassured that their dignity will be maintained at all times are of paramount importance.

The investigation environment

Working in a hospital for a long period of time can make it difficult to remember how frightening a place it is for most of the population. Older people who have enjoyed good health and never been a patient will not know what to expect and may just remember horror stories from their youth about the dreadful things that they believed used to happen in hospitals. Younger people could just be anxious about going into an unfamiliar environment and being obliged to submit their bodies to the ministrations of strangers. Children pick up on any negative emotions emitted by their parents.

There are a few key points that could be considered to help create a less threatening/more welcoming environment, taking patients' feelings into consideration. The first thing we must do is to think carefully about what to call the clinical investigation unit. A definition of a laboratory is 'a place equipped for experimental study in a science or for testing and analysis'. Even institutions with strong research priorities should consider exchanging this outmoded word for one more suited to today's more relaxed, patient-oriented environment. Patients are naturally worried enough about having to attend a hospital department without having to deal with the concern generated by an invitation to be examined in a laboratory. The word could be substituted quite simply with 'unit', 'department', 'suite' or even 'room'. Invitation letters can be helpful here and their wording should be carefully considered. Investigators will have different ideas about the type and amount of information to include in a letter and whether or not to enclose an information leaflet. Preference may be dictated by the nature of the investigation. Patients who are to undergo oesophageal studies receive an appointment letter as shown in Figure 11.1. There is quite a lot of information contained here because patients need to undertake several days of preparation and also understand what will be required of them during the 24 hours that the pH-recording device is *in situ*.

Conversely, it may be better to send a briefer appointment letter to the patient who is to have anorectal studies (Figure 11.2), which requires virtually no preparation and is over when he or she leaves the department that day. The main reason for this is that, should the letter go astray or fall into the wrong hands for any reason, the wording is ambiguous enough not to create any interest in anyone other than the patient and thereby cause him or her embarrassment. In the experience of the John Radcliffe Hospital, patients who have not already had their forthcoming investigations carefully explained by the referring clinician would either ring the department to ask or wait until the day of the investigation for a full explanation. By the same token, information leaflets should be distributed in the department only where their contents can be expertly described in a reassuring manner, rather than sent through the post and (frequently) not be read or understood and end up in the bin.

History taking (patient assessment)

It is not enough to ask a few basic questions before embarking on a series of physiology studies. It could be argued that the task can be carried out competently if all that is required by the requesting physician is a series of figures to assist in confirming a diagnosis; but it is much more helpful to conduct a thorough investigation by formulating careful questions and answers beforehand. This will also give the investigator time to gain the patient's confidence before embarking on actual studies. It may be that the initial interview before referral was a hurried affair as a result of time constraints or because the patient did not feel enough of a rapport with the clinician to volunteer key information. It is possible that the doctor was not particularly skilled in the finer points of history taking or, more frequently, that the patient felt guilty about 'bothering' the

Dear

Oesophageal Motility and 24-hour pH study

An appointment has been made for you to have this investigation here on:

Before the test

- Have nothing to eat or drink for **4 hours** before the test.

- It is very important to stop taking any of the following drugs **4 days** before the start of the test:
  Losec (Omeprazole); **Zoton** (Lansoprazole); **Protium** (Pantoprazole); **Pariet** (Rabeprazole); **Zantac** (Ranitidine); **Tagamet** (Cimetidine); **Prepulsid** (Cisapride). However, if you suffer intolerable symptoms after stopping the drug please contact me to discuss this on the number below.

- You may continue with antacids, eg Maalox, Settlers, Gaviscon, Rennies etc, until **24 hours** before the test.

- If you are taking medication for any other conditions, eg diabetes, epilepsy etc, continue as normal or telephone for advice.

Although you will not be sedated during this test (but local anaesthetic may be used if you wish) you **must not drive** a motor vehicle. Your insurance will not cover you. Please ensure that you are accompanied by someone who can drive you home.

You will need to return here 24 hours later to have the recorder removed, unless you wish to remove the device at home and return it by post: details for this will be given to you.

Female patients will find it more comfortable to wear a separate top and skirt or trousers so that the recorder can be worn under your clothes and around your waist. Further information is given over the page.

Additional information about the test

A very fine acid-measuring tube is passed through your nose and into your gullet. You should feel only minor discomfort from this (local anaesthetic gel or spray can be used if you wish). The tube remains in place for the 24-hour period of the test and is attached to a recording machine (rather like a Walkman) which is worn around the waist on a belt and removed the next day.

During the 24-hour period

Do

- Be as active as you would normally be, within reasonable bounds
- Go to work if you wish, providing driving or heavy manual work is not involved
- Eat and drink as normal, including food that may provoke your symptoms
- Record all symptoms on the diary card provided; this will be explained to you

Do not

- Drive a motor vehicle
- Take any medication for indigestion
- Take a bath or shower as the water may affect the data on the machine
- Chew gum

Contact number for information: 00000 000000 or 00000 000000 (bleep 0000)

Figure 11.1 Appointment letter for patients undergoing oesophageal motility studies.

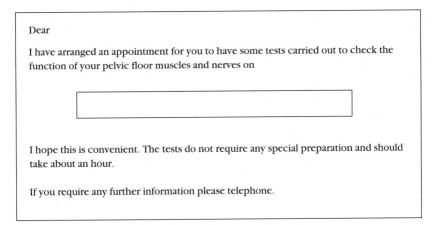

Dear

I have arranged an appointment for you to have some tests carried out to check the function of your pelvic floor muscles and nerves on

I hope this is convenient. The tests do not require any special preparation and should take about an hour.

If you require any further information please telephone.

Figure 11.2 Appointment letter for patient undergoing anorectal studies.

doctor with minutiae because 'Doctors are so busy and should really be spending time with someone sicker than me.' This is the most common misconception by patients who have been driven to desperation by the pain, discomfort or inconvenience caused by their symptoms to seek professional help, either because all home remedies or over-the-counter treatments have failed to give relief or because concerned relatives have insisted that medical help is sought.

Experience will create a sixth sense for detecting unexpressed but nevertheless anxiety-provoking concerns, and open questions should be asked to encourage further information. Years of expertise and intuition will enable a skilled history taker to recognize someone who is more inclined to chat about inconsequential matters than give direct answers to questions about their condition. There are those who may have 'verbal diarrhoea' or who are lonely and delighted to have the chance of passing time and engaging in conversation with a friendly person who seems to have time on his or her hands. Although it is essential to create a welcoming and friendly environment, it is also important to remain in full control of the situation and to keep an eye on the clock so that time is used economically and not wasted. This ensures that the patient gains full benefit from the time allowed for the interview and subsequent patients are not kept waiting. Conversations may be continued during the time that investigations are being carried out.

The investigator will need to know as much as possible about the patient's relevant medical (and, where appropriate, psychological) history, and patient records should be available and carefully read before taking a history. If they are not, and there is only a cursory request from a clinician for the investigation, then further information should be sought. Most doctors now realize the importance of this but, if the request is met by an unhelpful response from a clinician who is not conversant with the philosophy of holistic care (as opposed to just attending to the part that seems to be causing the trouble), an invitation to observe the department on a busy day will probably go a long way to improving this attitude. Doctors should understand that it is necessary to have as much information as possible to carry out the task efficiently.

Occasionally, the information given in a referral letter may conflict with what the patient considers to be the actual problem; it should be borne in mind that most patients know their own bodies, and the whole point of taking a history is to glean information from the patient. A quick phone call to the doctor may rectify any misunderstandings but, during careful history taking, the core of the problem is likely to be elicited anyway. It should go without saying that personal details – name, date of birth, address and hospital number – should be checked before any work begins. A skilled professional should not be content to carry out a requested investigation if it is quite clear that, because the correct questions were not answered at the time, another investigation, necessitating a further journey for the patient and possibly more unpleasant preparation (fasting, enemas, etc.), might be required. Every opportunity must be given for the patient to give as extensive a history as possible. Leading questions should be avoided, as many people would wish to give an answer to please.

The kind of questions to be asked, depending on the request and the policy of the department, should include – for both upper and lower GI investigations – the duration of symptoms, allergies, family history, height, weight, diet, previous surgery and medical conditions, previous investigations, and medication and its efficacy. For lower GI investigations details of bowel habit need to be elicited, including any changes, abdominal and urinary symptoms, and obstetric history when interviewing women (Figure 11.3).

The nature of the investigations should be explained as fully as possible to patients, giving them every opportunity to ask questions. The environment should be made as private and comfortable as circumstances allow – doors closed, curtains pulled, etc. – and the patient asked to remove the necessary clothing and lie on his or her left side, covered with a blanket if undergoing anorectal physiology studies. If upper GI investigations are to be

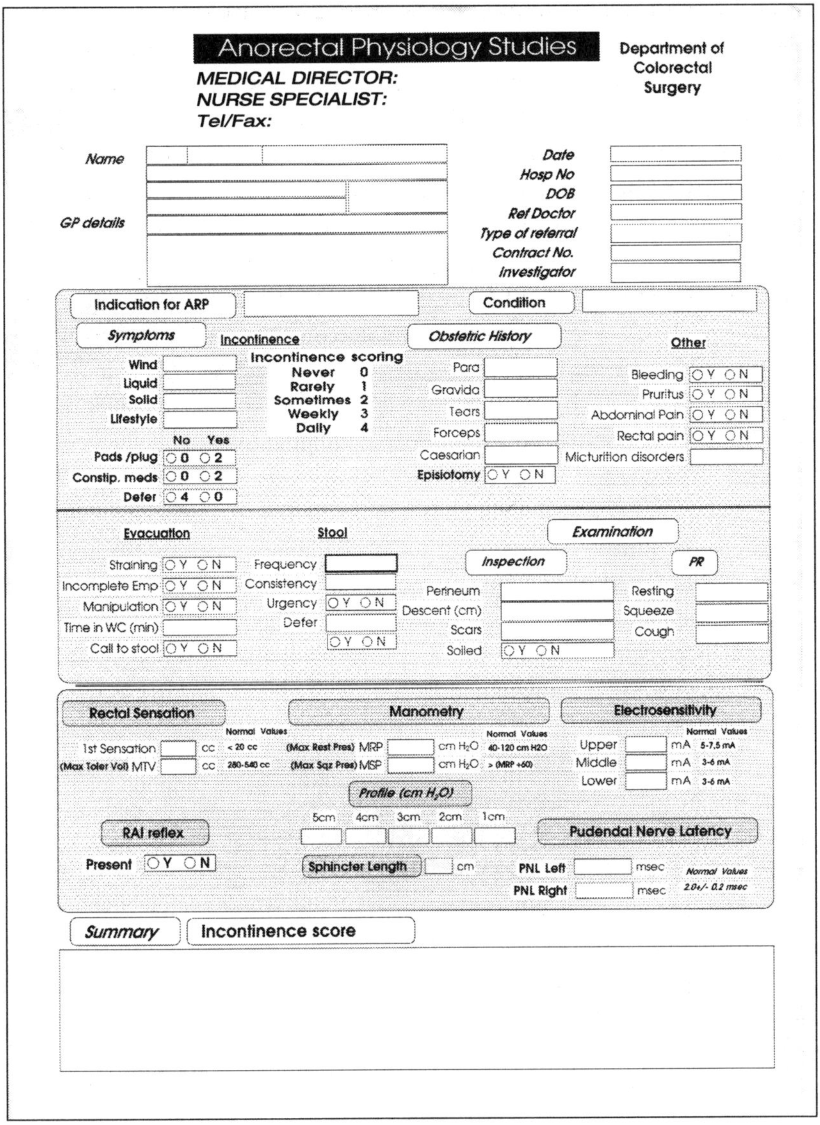

Anorectal Physiology Studies

Department of Colorectal Surgery

MEDICAL DIRECTOR:
NURSE SPECIALIST:
Tel/Fax:

Name

GP details

Date
Hosp No
DOB
Ref Doctor
Type of referral
Contract No.
Investigator

Indication for ARP

Condition

Symptoms

Incontinence

Wind
Liquid
Solid
Lifestyle

Incontinence scoring
Never 0
Rarely 1
Sometimes 2
Weekly 3
Daily 4

No Yes
Pads /plug ○ 0 ○ 2
Constip. meds ○ 0 ○ 2
Defer ○ 4 ○ 0

Obstetric History

Para
Gravida
Tears
Forceps
Caesarian
Episiotomy ○ Y ○ N

Other

Bleeding ○ Y ○ N
Pruritus ○ Y ○ N
Abdominal Pain ○ Y ○ N
Rectal pain ○ Y ○ N
Micturition disorders

Evacuation

Straining ○ Y ○ N
Incomplete Emp ○ Y ○ N
Manipulation ○ Y ○ N
Time in WC (min)
Call to stool ○ Y ○ N

Stool

Frequency
Consistency
Urgency ○ Y ○ N
Defer
○ Y ○ N

Examination

Inspection

Perineum
Descent (cm)
Scars
Soiled ○ Y ○ N

PR

Resting
Squeeze
Cough

Rectal Sensation

Normal Values
1st Sensation cc < 20 cc
(Max Toler Vol) MTV cc 280-540 cc

RAI reflex

Present ○ Y ○ N

Manometry

Normal Values
(Max Rest Pres) MRP cm H_2O 40-120 cm H2O
(Max Sqz Pres) MSP cm H_2O > (MRP +60)

Profile (cm H_2O)

5cm 4cm 3cm 2cm 1cm

Sphincter Length cm

Electrosensitivity

Normal Values
Upper mA 5-7.5 mA
Middle mA 3-6 mA
Lower mA 3-6 mA

Pudendal Nerve Latency

PNL Left msec
PNL Right msec
Normal Values 2.0+/- 0.2 msec

Summary

Incontinence score

Figure 11.3 Investigation of bowel habits: form.

conducted, an explanation of the procedure should once again be given and the patient made comfortable on the examining couch in the position dictated by the examining equipment.

It is often the case, particularly in teaching or research establishments, that students or visitors are present. Permission for this should always be sought from the patient before investigations are embarked on and, usually, patients are happy to oblige. It should never be presumed, as so often happens, that patients must be expected to tolerate the presence of extra personnel. Similarly, one should never talk over the heads of patients to students or visitors, but include them at all times. In this way the atmosphere in the room can be kept light and friendly, but professional. Maintenance of dignity is paramount. (This seems so obvious but lapses in correct behaviour happen all too frequently.)

When the patient has been made comfortable and a comprehensive history has been taken, the procedures to be carried out are carefully explained and then conducted according to the protocol of the particular department, reassurance being given throughout the time allotted to the tests. Not enough emphasis can be placed on the importance of communication in running an efficient and successful department. Courtesy titles should always be used when addressing patients unless they specifically request otherwise. The present fashion for using first names uninvited may sound harmless enough, but it is not desirable in such a sensitive environment and on the whole patients do not like it. There is plenty of anecdotal evidence to support this but, unfortunately, empirical literature is hard to find. A friendly yet professional atmosphere is the aim and this can be achieved only if the patient does not feel compromised in any way. Similarly, investigators ought to introduce themselves by their titles and surnames, and wear name badges prominently. Ideally, the investigation environment should be as private as possible in practice and, certainly, patients would not wish to be asked personal questions or discuss their symptoms where the conversation can be overheard. However, the physiology unit can be made to look less threatening with the use of attractive curtains, pictures on the walls and music playing softly. If the patient wishes for a relative or friend to be present this could be accommodated if there is sufficient room.

It would be helpful to arrange for as many tasks as possible to be performed at the time of the initial investigation. Much NHS time and money could be saved if two or three investigations were coordinated on the same day. Many people have busy working lives, but even if they did not they would still appreciate the opportunity to spend more time in one go, having a number of jobs done, than having to undertake the journey several times. A good example of this would be for an endoscopy, motility studies and barium swallow to be arranged to take place on the same day. This would cut down on travelling time, expense and worrying about organizing one's life to cope with another visit to the hospital. Another example is shown in a patient who has previously been investigated in the outpatient department for constipation or obstructed defecation, or faecal incontinence, who is then referred to the physiology unit for basic anorectal manometry to eliminate anal sphincter involvement. If doctors could be encouraged to request that anorectal physiology studies and evacuating proctogram – or anorectal physiology studies and flexible sigmoidoscopy – be conducted on the same day, this would be helpful to the patient and also encourage communication between departments.

Conclusion

Although we still have some way to go in the face of the 'old guard' being resistant to innovation, changes are definitely happening. The ideal situation, promoted by the Association of GI Physiologists (AGIP), which proposes accreditation of GI clinical measurement departments managed by registered physiologists, should soon become a reality. I believe that the most efficient departments will be staffed by interdisciplinary teams, each contributing their specific skills – scientists, clinicians, technologists and nurses who strive to achieve a balance of care which preserves patient dignity while undertaking prescribed physiological investigations. It is desirable, in this enlightened climate, that we should all learn from each other to create a more caring environment for patients and a more stimulating workplace for each other.

References

1. Kronecher H, Meltzer S. Der Schluckmechanismus, seine Erregung und seine Hemmung. Arch Anat Physiol 1883; 7: 328–362
2. United Kingdom Central Council for Nursing, Midwifery and Health. Final Report on the Future of Educational Preparation and Practice. London: UKCC, 1993
3. Finlay T. The Scope of Professional Practice: a literature review to determine the document's impact on nurses' role. NT Research 2000; 5(2)
4. United Kingdom Central Council for Nursing, Midwifery and Health. The Scope of Professional Practice. London: UKCC, 1992
5. United Kingdom Central Council for Nursing, Midwifery and Health. Code of Professional Conduct. London: UKCC, 1992

Index